Climbing Down Mount Everest

Climbing Down Mount Everest

My Struggle with Weight

Kirsten Crabill

Designed by David Crabill

Illustration by Molly Zak

ISBN 978-1466213104 (pbk.)

Printed in the United States of America

Printed by CreateSpace

Contents

Acknowledgments

I wish to express my deepest heartfelt gratitude to the following people whose kind assistance helped me with the writing of this book.

David, my dearest husband, who helped me bring this book to completion.

Thank you my friends for your skillful editing and genuine weight advice. Don Breitbarth, Eric Crabill, Martha Crabill, Perry Crabill, Donald Drucker, Ellen Figueira, Bobbi Fuhr, Anita Goldwasser, Sally Hayse, Eva Hess, Barbara Kyser, Edward Lee, Jenny Lee, Kyung Lee, Dee Marik, Julie and Jonathan Neri, Gary Pace, Rosemary Pericic, Beth Peterson, Charlotte Pflug, Laurel Renish, Michelle Schuster, Sue Stimack and Vikram Warraich.

Climbing Down Mount Everest

CLIMBING DOWN MOUNT EVEREST

Hiking On the Mountains in My Life

The last book I read was *Mountains Beyond Mountains*, a biography about Dr. Paul Farmer. He went to Haiti, Russia, Cuba and Peru to help cure the sick people of the world. He mentions a Creole quote: "Beyond the mountain is another mountain." This book isn't about him, but it is about me.

One mountain after another is the challenge of my life. No sooner have I made it down one mountain, I see another mountain before me that I need to conquer. Angel wings carried me from my father's arms in Germany to my mother's heart in Texas, over mountains and mountains of water. Strangers' hands were held out to me, while walking the mountains of China. A giant loving arm was held out for me to hold, while walking down the mountain to get home from Georgia. One mountain, which is always there, which is so difficult for me to conquer, is my own weight problem, my virtual Mount Everest. This one is the tallest! I've walked up and around it, but can't seem to get down the other side. This time, THIS TIME IT WILL BE DIFFERENT!

Sitting in my closet is a little orange stuffed animal named Nemo. I took my fish out the other day to look at him. I told him over and over that I am going to make it in my weight loss journey, which is one of the biggest battles of my life. He just listens and doesn't make any judgmental remarks. I am not even sure my husband believes I will succeed this time.

In school I was an average height and weight for my class. The teachers of my weight loss class are pencil thin, not even the width of a magic marker. Most people wish to be a pencil.

When I went to school, girls as thin as my teachers in weight loss class were laughed at. "Look at that skinny girl, let's not play with her!" The same was true for the fat girls. "She's fat; we don't want her on our team." So I grew up "normal." The only problem is, depending on a person's metabolism, her age and genetic inheritance, the normal person *either stays normal, can lose weight, or gain it. I feel I will be the only person, even after losing 50 pounds, who will still be in a size 1X.*

Mount Everest is 29,029 feet tall. In this book I plan to climb down Mount Everest. I will weave through (1) my life, including what I can remember on my diet and environment over the years; (2) notes from my weight loss class; *and* (3) my research on weight and other issues. *This is the tapestry of my life.*

A New Beginning

Fifteen students showed up for the first session of the weight loss class. We each received a workbook and were weighed. The teacher used a special scale to tell us our percentage of body fat. On my processing sheet, pencil woman number one wrote 50 percent body fat, and then opposite the number she wrote in her editorial comment, "V. Poor." The students walked over to pencil woman number two, who took their blood pressure. While waiting in line, I talked to four other people who stood behind me. Two were about the same weight as me or heavier and one was noticeably thinner. I told them that one of the results I would like by the end of the class is to have a "weight loss" friend whom I could talk to.

My turn came to sit and have my blood pressure taken. The nurse, pencil woman number three, struggled with my sleeve and then said, "It's okay, we will do it over your sleeve." She then remarked, "Your heart rate is very fast, are you upset over something?" I said, "Yes, never in my life have I been told that I scored 'Very Poor'." She didn't comment, so I started filling out their questionnaire. By the end of class, I hadn't completed the questions, which were supposed to indicate how motivated I was to lose weight.

Leaving Germany

This is my pre-history. By that I mean the part of my life that I cannot remember, but it is recorded in newspaper clippings.

The newspaper said,

> Baby Girl Flying Atlantic Alone to Mother in Edinburg (Texas) DALLAS – A two year old German girl is flying unaccompanied from Germany to Texas to join her mother, American Airlines said.
>
> Kirsten Huettig will arrive here at 5:10 p.m. Friday (June 17, 1948) on her way from New York to San Antonio. There she will join her mother Mrs. Eva Huettig of Edinburg, Texas.... Mrs. Huettig came to Texas in February 1948 after spending 30 years in Germany with her parents. She is an American citizen born in Washington State. During the last war she lived in Berlin. She moved to the

western zone of Germany when the Russians moved into Berlin. [Mutti told me about the 11-day walk at night to escape the Communists.] Her husband, a German citizen, is employed by the British military government at Buende, Germany. He plans to join his family in Edinburg in about six months. Mrs. Huettig is employed as a bookkeeper for the Hidalgo County News, a weekly Edinburg Newspaper.

Mutti, German for "mommy," and what I called my mother, cut out this article with no reference to the newspaper that it came from. Our family, one-by-one, got all the official papers needed to be American citizens. According to my mother, if at any time any one of us would have been denied our citizenship, we would have all returned to Germany.

Another newspaper article read:

"Confusing 5,000 Miles" A 2 year old girl who had traveled alone "all the way from Germany landed at Love Field...." Another article said, "Tears all German Tot Has When She Greets Mother." "Mutti, Mutti, Mutti," she cried over and over, not realizing that she was in her mother's arms. A bright red scooter, a new doll and a big cowboy hat failed to stop her tears. Once she broke away and went to M.

M. Davis of Charlotte, who had won her friendship in New York City and looked after her from there.

Mutti later told me that this lady spoke German and comforted me when I walked up and down the aisle crying "Mutti, Mutti, Mutti."

I was the youngest person to make this journey alone. I was the first. Life for me really began in Texas, close to the Mexican border. If ever anyone feels American, it's me. I feel extremely proud to be an American.

The First Five Pounds

At the next weight loss class, I saw a woman I hadn't seen before. She was in Class B, which was next door. She had gained some weight since her last class, and wanted to get it off. As she stepped on the scale she said, "I just found out I'm pregnant." A conversation ensued, and the weigh-in pencil said, "Oh, you don't want to gain any weight the first trimester." I imagine the woman's doctor had discussed her weight with her. I was told the same thing 37 and 34 years ago. The weigh-in pencil was trying to be helpful, as really you never know; perhaps the pregnant lady's doctor had not discussed weight with her.

Meeting this new lady reminded me of how all of the weight loss programs work. Victims full of anticipation join then can't hold to the regimen. After a few months they gain the weight back and voila – they have to dole out more money to re-join the weight loss program.

Next, it was my turn. I was going to keep my shoes on as I had forgotten how I had done it the first time. All I could remember is that I was second in line, and for the body mass index reading scale (percentage of fat) we had to remove our socks. My first thought was, "how unsanitary." As if she was reading my mind, the pencil scampered over to a bag and pulled out some disinfectant wipes.

Getting back to class, the pencil lady weighing me in said, "No, I remember you took off your shoes." Okay, so I did. This was a simple enough request. Next she noticed that I had a cotton long-sleeve lightweight jacket over my shirt. I said I wanted to keep it on because I was wearing just a cotton blouse, as the weather was 60 degrees and that next week it may be colder and I will wear a sweater. I felt it would make a difference in my weight. She was firm with me and said, "Oh, no it wouldn't." She insisted I take off my jacket before she weighed me. She knows the program. I knew I had lost several pounds and keeping the jacket on would not have destroyed my weight loss. She wasn't going to weigh me if I didn't take my jacket off.

The scale said I had lost 5.4 pounds. Other students gradually filed in to get weighed. The class started with another teacher reading some of the information in the workbook word-for-word. This week, the class size had shrunk from 15 to 10, with the heaviest five not coming back.

I told the lady at the scale that the instructions they gave us for losing weight said not to go on a crash diet. I told her that for me their diet was a crash diet. Obviously, she had never had a serious weight problem. She stood by her program "not being a crash diet." I explained to her that any large reduction in calories is a crash diet. I have no idea if she understood; she just stood there.

Struggling On the Mountain

It was and is a crash diet for me. Hopefully, by the end of the program, this will be the new way I eat, and the old diet will be finally over and buried. In fact, as I spoke to my diabetes support group about my weight loss, my face had a smile on it as I told them, but at home, where no one can see, tears of sadness come out of my eyes. I get melancholy thinking about it. I must bury my own eating habits, and the relief from the day, either joys or sorrows, will have to be met another way.

In the beginning of this diet I walked around like I was in detox. I could have been in the Betty Ford Clinic for an eating disorder. Technically, my disorder should be called "eating whatever you want, when you want" disorder. The ectomorph body type can do this and never gain weight. How lucky they are that they can really live. I do the other parts of my life with gusto, so why not eat with gusto? Never before, except for a job that I didn't like, did I watch the clock. You know, every second counts, like every calorie. I DO things. I don't measure every aspect. (One exception is when I make quilts.) I am losing some of my spontaneity and heading to robot land. How boring. The teacher says, "Dull is the new Thin." It is like chopping off a piece of me and I need to mourn. You better believe it. It HURTS. Why do I have to do this? I know why. I am getting too heavy. But being heavy didn't stop me from doing anything before. Being thin might. We shall see.

As to why I started the weight loss program this time, the 17th time, the answer is in this book. I know many people start over and over. Money flows from the heavy person's pocket into the program's cash register. In that moment, you feel you are a victim.

It's January; doesn't everyone start a weight loss program in January? All of you overweight people out there raise your hands. I can see most of them going up. On my own, I tried to eat almost nothing, but I got sick with a cold two days later. Lying in bed, I called a well-advertised weight loss program to see what it was about and get the cost. I thought it was too expensive, so I decided against it.

A long time ago, when my children were in Junior High School, my good garage sale buddy, Cathy, told me she gained the weight right back after she quit the program. I remembered that. But, when you are sick in bed feeling like a blimp, you are willing to try anything; even a program your friend once said let the weight creep right back on when she started eating the way she used to eat.

Getting started on a diet is the hard part. I was sick after two days on my own diet. I blew it. I drank a lot of orange juice, too much. This blew my already diabetic numbers to the sky. I got well after a week and looked into another plan that I had seen at another location. Then, a light bulb moment came. I would check to see if a local recreation center had the same program. It turns out that they did, so I jumped on it. I don't jump rope in my real life, maybe that exercise would have helped. I jump in my mind, and my mind will get the pounds off. Where I land after jumping off the high calorie trampoline into the world of the thin pencil people, who's to say? That's in God's hands. I'll do my best at doing my part.

I have been sick for two weeks now. The stress on my body has been severe. The first night after I began the weight loss program, I woke up at 2:00 a.m. My husband, David, was just coming to bed. I sat upright in bed, drenched with sweat, and asked for something to eat. I couldn't get up. David knows the drill, as this has happened before.

Every diabetic is different, just as every person is different. Some diabetics have a little warning when their blood sugar is getting low, but I am not one of them. The symptoms of a blood sugar "low" come on fast with me.

David went to the kitchen to fix the usual remedy. This is the one that works for me: a piece of bread with a large amount of peanut butter on it, covered by an obscene amount of jelly, and a glass of milk to wash it all down. The goal is to see how fast I can get the food in me.

The recipe is for jelly, the fast acting ingredient to raise my blood sugar first, followed by the peanut butter and bread, and last comes the milk, to cover the rest of the night. No one told me this, so I just made it up out of necessity. When I get like this, I am so out of it that I don't even enjoy what I am eating. The next morning I had to look at the jar in the refrigerator to see if it was marmalade or grape jelly.

People that live with gusto live all the way, including overeating and over medicating with food. When your car breaks down by the side of the road you don't request Chevron gasoline, you take whatever you can get and as much as you can get of it.

You just have one life, so take all you can get. Fortunately for me I have lived in several countries, and several states. If I could do it over I would take in more countries, more states, and more experiences. My life has not been less and less, but more and more. This is one of my psychological stumbling blocks with food. It was a joy to my life, and now the joy of eating is being buried by my own hand, and I mourn. What else am I supposed to do?

The Light of Wellness Shines on Me

Why should I start a new diet now, you might ask? Here's the reason: I have been having insomnia. I finally admitted to my husband about the sleepless nights. I could barely get up by 9:30 on most days. Daylight forces me to wake up. Then I "come to," but I really don't "come to" until about four in the afternoon, and then I feel like it's eight in the morning. And so the next night is the same way. After much soul searching I discovered what my problem was. It finally came to me. A few times at night I had felt my heart beat funny, just slightly off step. This caused me alarm, as once when I took a "physical" in Georgia the nurse said to me, "When you have to worry is when you are out of breath while resting." I was resting and I wasn't out of breath, but my heart wasn't right. I was afraid I was going to die, which was keeping me from going to sleep. I was tormenting myself. This was my brilliant idea: how to postpone death, just lose weight.

We have all read that mortality rates for overweight people are higher. We know this, but until we FEEL it, the impact is not real. I feel, I live, I lust for a rich life, only too rich has to be reduced calorie wise. That's my struggle. It's my life, or is it my rich life? Just existing is better than nothing at all. Where is the joy, the fun, and the extra energy when you are thin? I don't notice any of it with a five pound loss. Right now it is a sacrifice. It is a loss. I am hoping, at some point, my life will turn around.

Being sick with the flu doesn't help my mood either. As Scarlett O'Hara from *Gone* with the Wind would say, "Tomorrow is another day." Now, I'll just make it through lunch. Tomorrow is a long way away.

The Gym

I went to the gym to try the "recumbent" machine. My eye spied an instructor whom I had once taken a water exercise class from. I asked him to help me with the machine. He's a man I really admire. He was in a motorcycle accident, and when he speaks fast his speech is a little slurred. He is young, strong and resilient. Once, when I was in the pool, as he was walking around giving instructions to the class, I said in a very quiet voice to the lady next to me, "I have trouble doing that." The movement was walking sideways, crossing one leg over the other. When I looked up I saw his back, with his head turned looking at me, and he said, "Practice, Practice, Practice," as he walked. Now, he is someone who deserves lots of respect. Donald, I hope you read this.

I told him I needed to start on the easiest machine. We moved to another room. He took me to the "Sci-Fit," which is the easiest level machine that they have.

Calories count; get on the ball; two classes and three pencil instructors equals five pounds lost. Be structured. Don't just LIVE. It is that structure that I also fight. I'm not analytical. I'm not mathematical. I just DO IT.

A new e-mail came from our class instructor, challenging us to see how many foods we can find that have only 100 calories. This is a reasonable request. The next comment raised the hairs on my arm. They checked their computers and discovered I had not signed up for their exercise tracking system. The instructor could not find my name on the list of the computer users. Well, fancy that. She knows nothing about me. If my own husband has not been able to train me beyond Google and e-mail, why does she think I would do this for her? What makes them think I will get on the computer to record what exercise I do, so they can check up on me? I'm not losing weight for anyone but ME.

Long after I quit the gym, and long after the 10 week course is done, I'll be plugging away, doing the best I can. I won't be exercising more and more to work myself into injuries; I've already done that. I have more age, and more diet and exercise experiences *than many of those "thirty somethings with only 20 pounds to lose."*

If she says I will have to sign up to stay in the class then I will do it, but I will not record a single exercise that I do. I don't need to get set up with a trainer, with the additional expense. I just need to MOVE.

Obesity Surgery

Other weight loss options that could help me are the different types of obesity surgeries. These are options that I had looked to for a quick fix. I didn't research them too extensively until I started writing this book. Once at a garage sale, I bought some of the "fat clothes" (as the seller referred to them) from a very nice thin young woman. As I sit here I am wearing one of her sweaters, but you know what? Now this sweater is getting too big for me and I'll have to donate it with my other "fat clothes." The lady at the garage sale had gastric bypass surgery, and she was really happy about it. Another lady I met in a locker room said she didn't like the idea of these surgeries. She knew someone who had her hair fall out due to malnutrition.

I've always thought these surgeries were quick fixes. This attitude is true when you don't know all the details about the lap band or gastric bypass. As a fat person you think this is a sure fire success plan. You don't need to know if it is going to work in the end, because you feel it will. Look at Al Roker, NBC's weatherman. He had obesity surgery, and as I remember, I saw some hospital scenes where they were preparing him for surgery. Al Roker said it is not a "magic bullet." He said gastric bypass can help with weight loss, but it won't help with your emotional relationship with food.

Many people really enjoy eating. They eat when they are happy. They eat when they are sad. They eat when they are successful. They eat when they have failures. They eat when it is an overcast, cloudy, depressing day. They eat when they pack an oversized lunch to go to the beach on a beautiful sunny day. For many people life is always an occasion to eat, and that means really EAT.

I know this so well, actually too well. I don't like to admit this, but I was part of it. Al Roker did regain some weight after his surgery. He has to maintain his weight daily and watch his portions. I read that you can regain the weight just by nibbling on food all day long. It is not a magic bullet like most obese people think.

Gastric Bypass

The gastric bypass surgery divides the stomach into a small upper pouch and a larger lower pouch (the "remnant" pouch). (*Wikipedia*) There can be complications like leakage, stricture and ulcers. Also, the patient can, and probably will, end up with nutritional deficiencies. The doctors usually have the patients take vitamin and mineral supplements.

I could qualify to have this surgery because my body mass index is over 40. The surgery is meant to be a tool to help you, but then you must alter your eating habits. Your stomach becomes a very small pouch that restricts the amount of food you can eat at one time. You feel full eating this smaller amount of food. There can be complications to the surgery, like hemorrhage, infection and hernia. There is a mortality rate of 7 percent (for laparoscopic procedures) and 14.5 percent (for operations through open incisions) during the 30 days following the surgery. (Wikipedia.org Gastric bypass surgery.)

I heard that the doctors often put you on a special diet before the surgery, to see if you are a good candidate. The success results can be fabulous. A person can lose 65 to 80 percent of their excess body weight. This is why the lure to obese people is so strong.

I was surprised when I read that many people go through depression following the surgery. I know that I am depressed about the loss of many of my favorite foods. The article says that you can have muscular weakness and fatigue, all of which I am experiencing. It's important that people who consider this surgery change how they feel about food prior to the surgery. If they do not change, they will have a massive shock that can lead to depression.

The Adjustable Gastric Band

The adjustable gastric band is a different weight loss technique. It is a belt that is placed around the top part of the stomach. Again, I could qualify for this, as my body mass index is high enough. Many insurance companies cover it now. I saw a price of $8,900. It is less invasive than gastric bypass. Since no part of the stomach is stapled or removed, the patient's intestines are not re-routed. It seems like a less drastic way to go.

The newly created stomach pouch will hold about half a cup of food, (an unaltered stomach can hold six cups of food). The band can be adjusted, but you still have to watch what you eat, and the amounts you eat, for the rest of your life. After the adjustable band procedure is completed, the patient can only eat a few ounces of food at a time. This food must be thoroughly chewed, or the patient may vomit.

The way I am working on losing weight is the slow way. I am not forced to eat tiny portions by a man-made restricted stomach size, but I do eat much less than before. I have to watch what I eat very carefully. My mind now tells me "you can't eat any more."

I am intrigued about one thing. Bariatric surgery helps regulate blood sugar levels. The article I read said, "Seventy-five percent of type 2 diabetes patients who undergo bariatric [gastric bypass] surgery no longer experience symptoms and no longer require medication." I sure hope by getting my weight down I can cut down on my diabetes medication. Time will tell.

I had heard a long time ago that the gastric bypass could be dangerous. Some patients die on the operating table. Many years have passed since then, but once that "risk of death" has been planted in my brain, either correctly or incorrectly, it is hard to forget. Another point I have to consider is that I have had diabetes for 20 years, so I am a slow healer. It takes twice as long for a wound to heal on my diabetic body.

I will be the tortoise in the Aesop fable, "The Tortoise and the Hare." I am determined to crawl slowly but steadily in my new direction. Others that have surgery may beat me there, but I will get there. In my quest for progress and through my class, I will develop good habits. The Hare's magic bullet surgery doesn't assure him that he will win. Perhaps he will, but I will also win, despite my slow speed.

The Second Five Pounds

The next week I lost five more pounds. I noticed there were more students present in this class. Several of them left and went into Class B. As I was waiting for Class A to begin, I noticed there was a long table filled with various sandwich bags of food. We were to guess how many calories were in each bag. I felt like I was 35 again, at a Tupperware Party. If I could answer the questions correctly, I'd get a small plastic potato peeler, or some such trinket. I played the game just like everybody else. I got some right, and I missed some. It was a mixed bag.

The instructor talked about a local Mexican restaurant, and said they have a burrito that is 2,000 calories. That's way more than my daily requirement. She told us it is hard to measure pasta because of so much air space. Right on. These teachers know their calories. Out of the three bananas on the table, the middle one, which is seven inches long, is the one that qualifies for the "100 calories." I'm exacting when I knit or make a quilt, but I don't walk around in my daily life with a ruler handy to measure bananas.

Before the quiz, the weight loss rewards were given out. My name came up, and the teacher said, "Kirsten Crabill lost 5.1 pounds." While giving me my reward she said, "Wasn't that FUN!" I felt like screaming, "No" really loudly, but I didn't want to make a scene. I had worked very hard and used the determination of an ox. It has not been fun for me.

Sometimes I grieve for the foods I have lost. While the teachers have valuable information to share, I don't think their jokes are funny. Even young Florence, who sat two seats down from me, said under her breath, "I was irritable all week." I figure that is not the comment from a happy weight loss person, so I know I'm not the only one who feels the way I do. That's what I mean about the class. It seems like there is a lack of honesty about how we really feel.

Looking back at my notes, the teacher said many people reward kids with food. One example that comes to mind is from my own life. I followed the guidelines in *Toilet Training in Less than a Day*. It was a popular book in its day, some 40 years ago. For my son, I wore a pocketed apron and loaded the pockets full of orange candy circus peanuts. The instructions were to give your child cup after cup of juice so as to induce urination, and then reward him each time with a treat when he used the potty.

My son was trained after two hours. We started first thing in the morning, and then after lunch I decreased the number of times I gave the sugar treat and supplemented the accomplishment with a hug. We were both so proud at the end of the day. It worked. The next day we all resumed a normal life and he was using the child's potty. We only used diapers at night.

I would do it again, despite the comment made in class. When something works, you stick with it. I've lost 10 pounds so far. My motto is to do what I have to do to get what I want (but don't break the law).

After telling us that people reward children with food, the teacher said, "Food is not a reward; you eat to live." I should underline that three times because that's the truth.

The Beautiful Park

When we moved back from Georgia, I wanted to help my son reserve a special park for my grandson's birthday party. As we were not residents of that area, we asked a person who we thought was our friend to help us. We have known George for many years, but even knowing someone for a long time isn't always enough. He knew how important it was for me to reserve this park.

He signed the papers to be our sponsor, but three hours later he called and said, "I have buyer's remorse." He went into detail about how he didn't have the money to pay lawyers' fees and how the park was not enclosed. He worried that an outside kid could wander into our group, fight with a four year old, knock him down and give him a concussion. His paranoid fears continued—that kid would end up in a coma needing constant medical care for the rest of his life. Were we going to pay for that? Would our insurance cover it? On and on he went about the sky falling down on us and did we know if all the children had health insurance?

I don't know how George walks out of the house without fear that a meteor will fall on him. Finally David got on the phone to try to calm him.

When the call was over it was after 6:00 p.m. and I was hungry. And so a weight loss crisis began. I had no food prepared, and had no time and no stamina, as the disappointment sapped my body. With each step I labored over to the refrigerator. What was I going to do? I felt really bad, and really sad. The park of my dreams was to be a gift for my son and grandson. Also, I had to get some food really quick. It was approaching 6:30 p.m. and I really needed to eat. Here is what I did.

Tip # 1
Have some cooked vegetables within arm's reach in your refrigerator.

I ate the contents of the quart size bag of yesterday's cold cooked carrots. Only when I was halfway through did it occur to me to put the bag in the microwave. Have some vegetables within arm's reach, so when your will is broken you won't grab your husband's cookies. A disaster could have happened that would have thrown my train off the track, and it would have happened in a split second, as anyone who has tried hard at losing weight knows.

We found event insurance to cover the party. The ball is in George's court. If he doesn't feel safe about that, then I guess we will have to let our dream park go.

I'm better today, but last night I couldn't even concentrate on the lawyer story on television. They had two cases in one show, and I couldn't separate the two stories as to who was fighting and about what. The night was a wipe out. But I stuck only to my carrots and one glass of milk. This would have been a cake and pie occasion before. A second piece would have follow to insulate my sadness. Oh, I was really, really sad.

I trusted George, but he didn't trust us. Friends are people that do for and share with each other. They take people like George to the emergency room in the middle of the night. David didn't take him just once, but he took him several times. I don't know what George is going to say, but I bet he will decide that he wants to get out of the contract, even if we get event insurance to cover anything that might happen.

Despite disaster in my mind and heart, I didn't give in to food. In my heart, if a cake had been on the kitchen counter, I would have eaten a piece immediately, to soothe my pain. But the reality is that food is not a medication, like the teacher said.

It works just the opposite way in that it is like putting salt in a wound. That food turns into extra calories, which turns into FAT on your body. Beware of the golden treat, as there is a brutal invisible knife waiting in the cake to cut your weight loss progress. I've worked too hard to assassinate myself now, even though it has just been a few weeks. Beware of that antiseptic white cake, because it is a wolf in a frosted cape.

Tip # 2
Do Not Eat When People Upset You.

As I was lifting a spoonful of cold soup from a pot on the stove, I stopped two inches before my lips, but didn't eat it. Crisis after crisis for me seems to lead me to cold food. Be strong and do not allow frustration and aggravation to lead you to eat.

My son offered to purchase event liability insurance and have George as the first person covered on the contract. My son was also going to be on the contract. This million-dollar coverage was still not good enough *for George. I am sure if the President approved it, George would not find it acceptable. This could have been a way for him to give a gift to our family, but he is afraid that lightning will hit and he will be held responsible.*

Alcohol and Chocolate

The teacher talked about alcohol and how it limits your food consumption willpower. This results in your desire to eat more, as you have lost count of what you have already eaten. Alcohol is a saboteur that you can encounter on your journey to lose weight. She also talked about chocolate. The price of eating one little piece of chocolate is 20 minutes of exercise. Something that surprised me that the teacher said is that for a single hour of exercise we didn't need any nourishment except water. The hour of sitting listening to the lecture was up, and I walked to my car, which might entitle me to a "lick" of chocolate. I have not seen a calorie count for that, so I'll just let that lick go.

Childhood Adventures in Texas

When I was born I weighed only six pounds. It was right after the war and my mother suffered from food shortages in Germany. At the end of her pregnancy she weighed five pounds less than when her pregnancy began, and this with six pounds of me in her. She told me how she hated beans, because that was often the only food she had. Once she asked a farmer in the country for a single potato. He didn't give it to her. I have photos of my mother and father that show their gaunt, worried faces.

Some of my family lived near Seattle and had a couple of generations behind them in America. My mother's birth, in Washington State, once saved her life when she was in a line-up of people to be shot by the Russians. When asked where she was born she said, "Washington." The Russian soldiers thought she was from Washington, D.C. and thus I am here today writing these pages.

My memory starts from age five when I was living in San Antonio, Texas. I grew up an American. I waited on the corner at 6:30 p.m. on Saturday evenings with my father to buy a Popsicle from the ice cream man.

My mother and father both worked full time. Now every time I pass their photos double-framed together in the hall, I throw them a kiss and thank them for how well they cared for me. Our family believed in adopting the American culture. German was spoken behind bedroom doors concerning areas of my upbringing. We always spoke English together. America was OUR COUNTRY and Germany was behind us.

Here are examples of other families we knew who embraced American culture. One friend's family came from Russia and her father became really excited about his new country and the hot dog he ate at Coney Island. Another friend's family only spoke French at home, but the minute they left the house they switched to speaking English. In the 1950s, people rallied around becoming American. When they first came to America, my mother cleaned houses and my father, who received his doctor's degree in History and Philosophy from the University of Leipzig, worked on a construction crew. Later, they became managers of a motel. As time passed, they worked themselves up the immigrant ladder.

My father became the shipping and receiving manager of Sears and Roebuck, and my mother was a bookkeeper for Rosenberg Brothers, a company that sold dry cleaning machines and supplies. She needed a job and told the two Jewish brothers that owned the place to give her a chance and she would prove to them that she could do the job. Despite the history of the war, and all the "Kraut" hate, two good Jewish men gave my

German mother a chance. They are both dead now, and the company doesn't exist anymore. Wherever they are, I want to send them love and thanks for what they did for my mother.

Weight wise, I went from six pounds at birth to 120 pounds in the seventh grade. When I was a child, weight was not something that was important to me, so I have no recollection of my weight changing. I never paid much attention to what we ate at home for dinner. I do remember what we ate Christmas morning. We had brown and serve rolls that we dressed up with cold cuts, cheese, and jelly. This easy breakfast was good for my parents, as they had stayed up late wrapping presents for me for Christmas morning. I cannot remember what we had for breakfast the other 364 days of the year.

One incident that I can remember involved a boy who also lived in the apartments. He would dig a hole in the dirt, fill it with sugar, and then wait for the ants to come before he drowned them with water. I didn't think this was funny. I knew it was wrong, even though I had never been given any instruction on how to care for animals. The apartments where we lived never allowed animals, so I never had one.

After witnessing this, I eyed the girls across the street even harder. I stood there and sadly watched them. I asked my mother to take me across the street so I could introduce myself to them; and they became my constant playmates. There were four girls, the oldest was my age, and the second oldest was just a year or two behind. The two others were "babies." We played mostly outside, except on rainy days. Often we climbed our favorite tree, and we sat there for hours feeling like kings, until it was time to eat lunch.

Our crowning masterpiece was created when we were allowed to play on a patch of dirt. We built a village there. We built small-scale houses out of blocks. We already had little cars and trucks. We drew roads in the dirt by using the side of a wide block. Many of the people in our tiny village were rich, so we created swimming pools out of inverted lids of mayonnaise jars. We made an entire town this way, and we did it over and over. The fun was in the creation, not in playing with it. It took us all day to build a village, and then it was time for me to go home. I used to love this even more than sitting in the tree or cutting up a refrigerator or washing machine box to make a house for the "babies" to play in.

Childhood Food Memories

Years went by and my most pronounced food experience was each Friday night we went to Piggly Wiggly to buy our groceries. We had no babysitter so I had to go along. My parents told me to be good in the store, and then they would buy me a doughnut. I stood by the glass-enclosed bakery counter for the full time they were shopping, trying to figure out which one I wanted. I was always good and I was always rewarded. My parents didn't have lots of extra money to reward my good behavior with toys, and thus came to be my wonderful memory of doughnuts.

Another food memory occurred when I was five. Even though school was out for Christmas break, I was still at the school for daycare because both my parents worked. Every year, on the afternoon of Christmas Eve, my mother would come to pick me up early after 1:00 p.m. from the daycare. We had to take a nap after lunch, and were all in an auditorium where there were rows of cots lined up for afternoon naps. We were supposed to have our eyes closed, so whenever I heard the teacher's footsteps coming in my direction I would quickly close my eyes. I never did sleep. The hour that I had to wait seemed like an eternity.

The excitement lay ahead after my mother picked me up. She was in charge of going to the local deli and getting the food for the Christmas party at work. At the deli I was eye-high to rows and rows of sliced meats, potato salads, deviled eggs, and other deli food I couldn't quite identify. There were more types of cheese than I ever knew existed. My eyes could see nothing else, just a long glass cabinet full of unlimited food, even beyond my sight. I had never seen so much food in all my life. When we left both of Mutti's arms were full of bags of food for the party. She had a hand free to hold mine as we walked down the city streets to her work. I was really feeling "important" as if I was the one in charge of the whole party.

Once at her work, all the food was laid out on a counter above my head, and like the others, my mother helped me to have a good lunch. Gifts were exchanged in a gift draw, and then we went home. The next day was Christmas, and another wonderful treat filled day. My dearest Aunt Iris always sent me gift boxes from Germany filled with chocolate every year of my life until she died. She loved me so much and this is how people in the 1950s showed love. Like mothers wearing aprons standing in the kitchen serving hot apple pie to their family. This was the American and German way. The terrible war was over, and now people had more, and it was time to share what we had with each other and enjoy it.

My American Aunt

Aunt Pamela told me about the side of our family who relocated to Washington State. World War II was hard on them. She said her mother had ration stamps for meat, butter and gasoline. Aunt Pamela told me how she had just started to drive, but she and her sister often decided to take the bus to save on their "gasoline allowance."

Their family lived in the country. With the help of a neighbor, her brother plowed a half-acre and planted a vegetable garden for the family. Coming out of the depression, life was difficult, and it was hard for her to forget those days. When she was in high school, she picked berries to make money for clothes to wear to school. Her mother received a "mother's pension" because her father had died a month before another sister was born. Aunt Pamela claims that the maternal "Venator" traits came out strong in both of them.

Her grandfather, Mr. Venator, owned a silver and copper mine in Austria-Hungary. He was a strong and robust man who lived into his 80s. He took his granddaughter ice-skating one afternoon, then took an afternoon nap and never woke up.

Aunt Pamela's mother stayed up nights making care packages for others in the family in Germany who were less fortunate. My mother told me about the beautiful baby clothes she received. They made her cry. These gift boxes were sent as soon as it was deemed "safe" to send packages to Germany.

Aunt Pamela's sister-in-law came from Graz, Austria. I saw the trunk that she brought to Ellis Island stored in her garage. Before Aunt Pamela was born, when her brother was three years old, he came over from Germany with his parents. Years later, there was no money for the young man to go to college, so he got a job working for the railroad at the Tacoma station. Afterward he met the young lady from Graz, and they were married.

At his home he tilled the soil and had perfect, straight rows of crops. He and his family fared much better than the urban population, and like my aunt says, "We were Upper Poor." With her mother and sister, she walked several blocks to a store and bought a five-cent candy bar that they split three ways.

They never had weight problems. My mother told me that her mother, and Aunt Pamela's mother, who were sisters, served big meals. To keep their weight down, they fasted one day a week. They didn't eat low calorie foods and stick to only 1,200 calories a day. They had families to feed and couldn't focus on modern day diets.

Aunt Pamela said there were a lot of war brides, German women who married American soldiers. The war severely affected so many people's lives. Aunt Iris's husband just vanished somewhere on a battlefield, never to be heard from again. She had a daughter who was born in an air raid shelter. Another one of her sisters was married to a Jewish man who apparently met a tragic end, although details about that incident were never discussed.

In Germany during the war, the soldiers were the first to be fed and the civilians the last. After my mother passed away, I opened her freezer to find foil wrapped cooked food filling every shelf from top to bottom. Six years of hunger during the war had left its mark on her. She told me that Hitler told the German people that the war was going to be only six months long, but instead it was six years.

In America during WWII, the war industry was humming. Aunt Pamela said that Henry Kaiser was building a ship a day. There was so much military activity around where they lived in Washington State; she often thought they were lucky they were never attacked.

Where Aunt Pamela lived, in the country, there were five houses along a one-mile stretch of road. Her family and her siblings rented 40 acres from the state. Later, when given the opportunity, they bought the land, and divided it between the families. There was a footpath that had been beaten down between the two houses, where I played one summer when I was 11 years old.

Another aunt sent Aunt Pamela's family $25 to buy a cow. They milked it to provide for their family. They also had some chickens. They made and canned applesauce from their apple tree. Prepared foods were just beginning to enter the market, but they had no money to buy them, and no reason to. They were growing their own food. She remembered Spam, which was new to them, although it was a staple in the American soldiers' diet. She heard it was popular in Hawaii. She is the second person that told me that. This second person has a brother that lives in Hawaii so I guess she should know.

In "elite" diet-conscious circles, canned meat is not acceptable. The food from a vegetable garden is "in." The problem is how many people have backyards large enough to include vegetable gardens, or have the time to plant and maintain them? There are some who do, but that way of life really no longer exists.

When Aunt Pamela was first married, she moved for a short time to Illinois. That is where my cousin was born. When my Aunt was 23 she would walk to the post office and stop off at the "sweet shop." She didn't drive like we do today. Aunt Pamela's mother walked a mile to work at a local school cafeteria to prepare food for the children's lunches.

After the family relocated to Washington, Aunt Pamela said they were never flush with money, and they primarily lived off their corn crop. They had enough to eat but there were not a lot of leftovers. She told me that our lifestyle today has led to our own "detriment." Both her daughter and I have diabe-

tes. Aunt Pamela thinks this is due to the fact that a lot of babies born after WWII were fed a formula of carob and corn syrup with evaporated milk. Corn syrup is now cheaper than sugar, although I don't know what the price was then.

Tip # 3
I Have Met Three Sharp Pencils!!!

This is a comment about the thin "pencils" teaching the weight loss class. These leaders are very sharp, although my first impression of them was upsetting when they wrote the note about my body fat. Make no mistake, these "pencils" are really sharp, and if you can get into a class with instructors like these, consider yourself lucky. They are knowledgeable pencils, of the best quality, but some of their remarks stab like a sharp point. I don't think they like me as much as some of the other humorous types. I am too serious for them. They are very knowledgeable, and I am soaking it up like a sponge. Get into a class taught by these three pencils and you can erase your fat.

One Thousand Jumping Jacks

There were only seven people in the class today. Irving has already lost 10 pounds, and he thought maybe he would get recognized. He is my nearest competitor. I've lost 12 pounds and I could make it a race with him in my mind, but why? Why am I doing this? The truth is

I want to lose as much weight as I can, and he can take care of himself.

Irving says he eats between working on projects at home. This is his pause and boredom break. It is just a habit that he has. I like his sense of humor, maybe some of it will rub off on me.

The pencil told us there are subtle cues from childhood, as when you were young and behaved well, you got a cookie as a reward. You felt good when you ate it, so the next time you accomplished a task, you looked forward to another cookie. In my case, you need to substitute doughnut instead of cookie.

As I'm sitting here with my husband across from me at the kitchen table, I see that he has a handful of peanuts. I told him that he needed to do 1,000 jumping jacks to combat the effect of those peanuts. He laughed at me and ate them all. What a killjoy I have become. As he left the house I said, "I could do 1,000 jumping jacks for you to combat those peanuts," and he laughed and said, "Yes, you could do that plus also get a trip to the hospital." For me, accomplishing this task could be written up in *Ripley's Believe It or Not.*

Florence, a class member, mentioned that she has a strong problem at that "time of the month." The pencil said that it is a craving that is hormonally driven. She told us you have two solutions when you are in a difficult food situation. You can either change your world or you can change your behavior. This philosophy specifically addresses the issue that I have about going out to eat. For me, eating out derails the train. I don't recover from the joy of eating wonderful food and I don't bounce back. The train just stays off the track and wants to continue to enjoy the wonderful food. It is like wanting to go to the deli, and being sure to stop off at the bakery for all the cakes you want so that you can continue the joy of eating delicious food.

In an e-mail, the pencil said either avoid going out to eat or go online and decide in advance what you plan to eat from the menu. Then, go to the restaurant and get the take-away box before you eat. (I used to get the take-away box at the end, but didn't have a lot of food to put in it.) She told us to ask the waiter to put all the sauces on the side and to not bring the chips or the bread to the table. Here is where I have trouble. I like the bread. These "being strong" restrictions take the joy out of eating, so I say to myself, "Why am I even going?" The joy of really eating has to be given up forever for me, as the first delicious meal derails the train. The pencil, as you can see, is trying to help us. Thank you, pencil.

Diet Soda

The pencil also talked about the detrimental effects of diet soda on some people. In an article about Diet Soda, Wikipedia says, "Forty-eight percent of the subjects were at a higher risk for weight gain and elevated blood sugar." Wikipedia goes on to say, "Drinking diet soda more than likely will increase cravings for sugar flavored sweets.... Animal studies suggest that artificial sweeteners cause body weight gain, theoretically because of a faulty insulin response, at least in cattle and rats." If I was a cow, I guess I would be in deep trouble. The diet drinks are my only sweet. I am now living a restricted dietary life, and I like the fake sugar. It makes me feel good, especially since caffeine is included in the mix.

Wikipedia goes on and says, "Rats given sweeteners have steadily increased caloric intake, increased body weight, and increased adiposity (fatness)." My calorie intake has gone way down, even with the diet sodas. I guess the rats like the fake sweet and want to eat more and more food. Right now I need the diet soda as a crutch. I feel I really need it. Maybe later I can let it go, but it gives me a lift and it is the one food joy that I have left.

The instructor then asked about the triggers that cause our problems. It was Alice's turn. She told the group that she tends to watch television and eat. She also said that she was depressed about her husband's death. She cried for a moment and the room was silent. After some talk about eating with the television on, the instructor said, "You know you can't replace your husband with TV and food."

I know what she meant, but it is a very sad thing when a loved one dies. Under such stress you do whatever you can to ease the pain. My criticism is that the teacher should have said: "I know this is a hard time for you, maybe you can listen to some music, or see some friends, or work on a project. Do anything that would keep you from eating." The pencil is young, and she has probably never experienced death.

Korean Sunshine

Yesterday I went to visit one of my best friends. Sunshine is Korean, and we first met when our sons were in high school. For many years we weren't close friends, but that has changed now. We visit when we can and share our lives together.

Both she and her husband are thin. I asked her to be completely honest with me, and tell me what she thinks about fat people. Before WWII, and through the Korean War, Sunshine said the Korean people thought fat people must be rich, and that is why they could eat so much food. There was a lot of poverty in Korea during that war, so it is easy to think that way.

After she came to America and food was more plentiful, there was one thing that came to Sunshine's mind when she saw fat people, and it has to do with her family history. She knows that obesity can cause diabetes. My friend is very aware of the link between being overweight and diabetes, so after she came to America and prosperity was slowly returning to the world, Sunshine told me that when she sees a fat person, the first thing that she thinks about is the link between being overweight and having diabetes.

Sunshine has two brothers. One didn't take care of himself, and before he died he was in a nursing home for 11 years. He ate all types of sugary foods, and when he went to parties, he conveniently forgot that he was diabetic, and eagerly helped himself to generous servings of cake. He was a normal weight for his size. One day he fell in the snow. His head was bleeding. He didn't get treatment right away at the hospital, as there was a more seriously injured person ahead of him. A month later he went into a coma. He lost all of his mobility and was wheelchair bound because of his brain injury. All of this was because he went out in the Wisconsin snow wearing only slippers, and slipped.

Sunshine's other brother, who lives in Hawaii, has been a diabetic for 35 years. He takes insulin and walks every day. He watches his diet and is not reckless when it comes to eating. Sunshine says this brother survived by walking. It is interesting that his daughter, who is a doctor, chose the field of diabetes to study. I suppose by going this route, if there were ever any breakthroughs, she would know and be able to help her father.

After discussing many more things in our lives, it was time for me to go home. Here is what she said while holding my hand:

Tip # 4
"Friendship lasts longer than Chocolate."

Sunshine is so right. Chocolate disappears in your mouth in seconds, whereas friends last for years. Bless her; she is really special to me.

My Difficult Journey

My trek down the mountain is getting hard now. The first 10 pounds were easy. The next two were difficult and the results were not nearly as spectacular. I have to chip through the hard ice now.

This morning I am watching a neighbor with his saw in his driveway through the window. I hear the motor running, and then plop, a small piece of wood falls on the ground. The thought came to me. How easy would it be for me to just go over there and submit myself to that machine? In only a minute, a large chunk of fat from my stomach or buttocks would land on the ground. A more refined process is for people to see a doctor who does body sculpting. I'm not trying to be a perfect Miss America; I'm just trying to chip away at this hard ice ahead of me so I can get to softer ground. I must persevere. Even though I have been working on it for almost four weeks, I have struggled too hard to let my progress evaporate.

Last night I was hungry at 7:00 p.m. My dinners are light in calories, maybe too light. I had exhausted the "calling a friend," technique, and didn't have the strength for another "morning walk," so I decided to sit in a hot bath. The hot water is very relaxing to me, but it does flare up the pain that I sometimes have in my left shoulder. When it becomes too hot for me, I get out, dry myself, and sit in the dark with a towel wrapped around me. My whole body relaxes.

I could feel the sweat coming down from my forehead, and I was thinking how these streaks of sweat were like the tears of my soul. My body was relaxed, but my mind was crying for all the Herculean effort I must take to reduce my weight. Some might ask, "Why are you doing it, if it makes you feel so unhappy?" I have to do it because I know that it is either losing weight or having drastic health issues ahead. Heart and knee problems are two things I can think of quickly. I am

STRONG, but underneath this strength, I also cry.

Happy Valentine's Day

I asked my husband for some flowers yesterday because I can't have chocolates anymore. Neither can I have the joy of going out to a nice restaurant, because all of the wonderful-tasting food will make me want to eat. Thin people can eat. This is a jealousy I feel. It makes me sad. Why can't I be the thin person who can eat all that food? I will be thinner someday, but I'll never be able to eat "all that food" without paying a horrific price at the scale. In class, Florence said that when she sees another person at a party eating more food than she could, she feels the unfairness of the situation: "Why can't I eat that much?"

"Why do I have to be hungry for an hour before lunch?" For some reason the water exercise class today was harder than I expected. I got out early even though I was enjoying myself. I drove home and was lagging in energy, wondering how I was going to hold up for another hour until lunch. David suggested we modify the mealtime and go get a fast food salad earlier than usual.

We were out the door in five minutes. I was painfully aware of how long it was taking the clerk to get my chicken salad ready. Then, once opening the plastic bowl, I found the chicken to be hot. He was heating my food, which accounted for the delay.

After this light lunch, we went to the drugstore and purchased another notebook for me to continue my writing. Next, we were off to Target to get a CD holder. We didn't like their selection, so David drove us to Fry's Electronics to look at what they had. He went in the store for me, as we had discussed what I wanted.

As I sat in the car, I was studying a map of Europe, and I was thinking how I would love to go to some of the cities near the Arctic Circle. Then I stopped thinking this when I realized I had trouble after just one hour of exercise. There is so much that I have done in the past, but when I was short of energy, I had extra food to eat. Now my fuel for each day lasts two-thirds of the day. I need to be home reading after that. Just to go to the class at 5:00 p.m. I have to push it. Do thin people run around with just enough energy for two-thirds of the day?

Just beyond my notebook is a clear vase with a red bow that holds twelve budding roses, with white baby's breath and green foliage. It is beautiful and I am happy I got this Valentine's Day gift.

There's a can of peanuts sitting on the counter. I've not had any for weeks. I broke down and had one, and shortly after that I wanted another one. I savored the first one. This is my problem, I simply enjoy eating. Food tastes so good, and just one bite or one spoonful makes me want more. Instead of having a second peanut I took the can and placed it on top of the refrigerator.

Does Eating Equal Happiness?

I told a friend, whom I hadn't seen for a while at the gym, that I had lost 12 pounds. She lit up and was all smiles. She noticed I wasn't joyful and asked me how I was doing. I told her the truth, that I was glad I had lost the weight, but that I wasn't happy. Whereupon she said, "Your happiness is in the food you eat." That is not entirely true. What I need "to feel well" is actually more calories, but more calories will make me fat. So each day I run around with two-thirds of a tank of gas to make it through the day. The last third of the day I run on fumes.

It's 3:30 p.m. and I've just eaten my second dill pickle. I can use a little extra strength, even if they don't have many calories. One thought crosses my mind over and over. John Adams, our second president, has written about his studying law at night while teaching school during the day. In a letter to a friend, He said:

Tip # 5
"It will be hard work, but the more difficult…the enterprise, a higher crown of laurel is bestowed on the conqueror…."
–John Adams

I want that "higher crown of laurel" for myself. No one will ever see it, but I will know it's there. I have not fought this hard to fail.

Grade School Thoughts

Where I stopped talking about my life was in San Antonio, and how I enjoyed playing with my four girlfriends. My parents were looking for a nicer apartment. I had told them about the boy who drowned the ants. Living above us were a husband and wife who were often fighting. The lady would come down the steps and each month it seemed like a different part of her body was in a cast. Once it was her leg, then it was her arm. I was perplexed at what was going on, as this was not how we lived. My mother told me the husband was hitting his wife.

When we found another suitable apartment we moved a block away to San Pedro Street. This apartment was nicely furnished with Rattan furniture. In my eyes, it was elegant. I was in fifth grade and could walk the one block alone to visit my four girlfriends.

The sixth grade made an impression on me for a few reasons. My teacher, a harsh teacher whom all of the fifth graders were afraid of, taught me something that no other teacher ever had. Her words of wisdom were, and I shall never forget them, "No one knows everything; the important thing to know is how to get the information for what you need to know." She taught us how to use library resources and how to understand maps. She opened up my world.

On the unpleasant side of the sixth grade, I was always one of the last ones standing when the team captains picked whom they wanted for their teams. Although I was average size and weight, I was not of average athletic ability, and was made painfully aware of it by being one of the last ones chosen. My memories about being in left field are ones of being thankful that I was there. For several months I had whooping cough, and always tried to hide it in the classroom, but in the field, with my other teammates far away, I could cough and cough until I felt like I was coughing my insides out.

That covered the first half of sixth grade. Then in the spring, several of us "average" girls were jealous of a "well-endowed" girl. Who would have ever thought that average wasn't good enough? The girl that I am talking about had a very large bust for her age. We noticed that the boys were giving her a lot of attention. The average girls, including myself, formed a plot against the budding beauty and buried her sweater. All of us got a "U" in deportment on our report card. That "U" stands for unsatisfactory, and was the only "U" I ever received. The teacher made us all contribute to have her sweater professionally cleaned.

In the summer after sixth grade, I went to Camp Idlewild, somewhere in the Texas Hill Country. There, the talk at dinner was that Alaska was to become the largest state, but that Texas was still the best. I remember we had to take salt tablets with our lunch because of the heat. After being there a day or two my swimsuit ripped, so the camp counselor called my mother who mailed me a new one. Who knows if I had a weight problem then, or if the suit was defective? I was just a kid and no one ever considered the fact that maybe I was a little fatter than before, or just a matter that I was growing into a larger size.

Life changed for me in the seventh grade. I asked my parents for a "sack" dress and got a red and white checkered one. This was the first dress I can remember in detail. Of course there were other dresses before, but body image and fashion, other than being "average," weren't important to me. I remember how my father drove me around all Saturday to get a gold "K" necklace. It was the rage of that year to wear a necklace that had the initial of your name on it. About four in the afternoon we finally found a place that had a "K" in stock.

Seventh grade is the first time I became aware that I weighed 120 pounds. Somehow, I had advanced from six pounds at birth to 120 pounds. I was aware of my weight for the first time in my life.

I didn't think about weight at all when our family went out to a little local Mexican restaurant and had hamburgers. I had one, and I didn't speak up to say, "No mayo please." It really didn't matter. I ate a whole one, bun and all. My weight was a number on one side of the page, and my food consumption was a totally different entity on the other.

The days in Texas were coming to a close as a major move was ahead of us, but first I had my summer vacation in Washington living with my relatives.

The Vegetable Garden

The rural life in Washington was completely different from what I had known in Texas. My Aunt Melissa always cooked fresh food from the garden that her husband tilled and worked on when he wasn't at his railroad job. He also made his own beer. It seemed like laundry was being washed in the washing machine out on the covered back porch every few days.

The evening meal was always a magnificent display of several bowls of food, more than we ever had on our Texas table. It was home cooked food, much of which came from their garden. I was aware that the food really did taste good, not fully realizing that much of it was the homegrown vegetables. Both of my parents worked, whereas my Aunt Melissa stayed home and had time to cook delicious German food.

Food was not a part of my life then. I did like how, at the end of a full day of play, we all sat down at the large round kitchen table. This table was off to one side and directly opposite a wood-burning stove. My aunt had two stoves. One was wood burning and the other was more modern and was used for cooking. This impressed me, as in Texas we only had one stove.

Sitting at the table, I could look out the window and see the vegetable garden. This was a pleasant sight, especially when the grown-ups drifted into adult conversation that didn't interest me. I really liked looking at the rows of corn and other vegetables. Sitting at that table eating dinner with them was a very special memory for me. After dinner the children never had to help with cleaning the dishes.

Our childhood was on "easy street." One fond memory was when a cousin, whose birthday is close to mine, would come over and we would all play in the woods between the two houses that were on the 40 acre lot. She and I were best buddies. We both had a crush on a boy cousin who was several years older than us, but he would have nothing to do with us. We played away our days. That was my Washington State summer vacation.

Teenage Years in Maryland

I flew from Washington to Maryland right before the beginning of eighth grade. My parents had driven from Texas to Maryland and found us a place to live. Not aware of my weight, but aware of boys, I finally began noticing them as "different." They were no longer just other sexless people on this earth.

My parents rented a house in Kensington, Maryland for a few years. Here is where one taste of reality hit me. No longer could I just sit and look cute in the classroom as I had done in Texas schools, I actually had assignments to look up 20 words in the dictionary, write their definition, and use them in a sentence. I thought I had graduated from seventh grade and gone directly to college.

I was required to take home economics classes, the first of which was sewing. In seventh grade in Texas, I labored through making a simple rectangular apron with a string tie for the waist. I struggled with a treadle sewing machine, where many of my stitches were uneven. I had a giant disappointment at the end. During the last step, I scorched the apron while ironing it. My grade at the end of this class was a C.

With much trepidation I entered into an eighth grade home economics class in Maryland. This time I discovered I was the best seamstress in the class. What changed? We had electric sewing machines.

In ninth grade I took Algebra 1, and it was there that I met my good friend Maria, whom I still have a friendship with after 50 years. We still laugh together when we think of the teacher who once wrote on the chalkboard: "I know I have a rip in the back of my pants." All of us giggled during that class. Both of us also knew the girl who was pregnant and had to leave school. Actually, that was the scandal that I remember. Never once did I focus on weight. In fact, it never even crossed my mind.

By the summer before the 10th grade my parents had saved enough money to buy a house. Remember that when they came from Germany they did not have many possessions. The concept of starting over in your 30s or 40s is something that was lost on me until I was an adult. This is very hard to do. Because the house was in Rockville, I could no longer go to the high school where my friend Maria was going.

I remember wishing we could have bought a house on the other side of the tracks, where the big beautiful trees were. There was a park over there, and I often went up there to relax and swing under the canopy of the big trees. At one point, after 11th grade, I had to take summer school, which is where I met my first boyfriend.

Here is where a very pronounced food memory comes in. Each day, after my political science class, I took the bus home. From the Rockville Turnpike bus stop, I walked through old Garrett Park, where I had wished that we could buy a house. I would wind through the streets until I got to the little store near the train tracks. Crossing the tracks, I would descend the hill to get home about two o'clock in the afternoon. After getting home, I always fixed myself a cup of Minute Rice. I didn't know how to cook real rice, but Minute Rice was easy for a teenager. After I waited the five minutes, I put on a heaping spoonful of butter and salted it with a few shakes of my fist. Then I enjoyed my late lunch. I don't know why I remember this; except that it was something I prepared myself. Still, I was never aware of how fat or thin I was, and I thought of myself as just being "average."

Sadness in a Young Heart

Tragedy struck at the end of the 12th grade when my father died. The day after he died I went out and got a job. Only I knew that he had wanted this for me. My father and I had talked about it. Some neighbors criticized me for this.

The plan was to get a summer job before attending Frostburg State College. I chose the University of Maryland instead, because it was cheaper. My mother tried so hard, and worked so hard. Until I was 18 we received some money from Social Security, but it was only for a few months, and not enough to really help us. Fate worked for me. My father's death forced me to attend another university where I eventually met the man I married.

My father was very special to me, and famous in that he was one of the few survivors who walked away from the bombing of Dresden in February 1945. The Allies did an extensive bombing of Dresden that caused a massive firestorm throughout the city. From

February 13 through February 14, 1945, between 35,000 and 100,000 people were killed.

Another famous man died a year before my father died. Most people will recognize his name. What happened to him was a major shock to our country.

I will start this part of the story by talking about walking down the hill from "old Garrett Park" to get to my house. At the top of the hill was a little store that had a pay phone. It was from that store at 3:00 p.m. on Friday, November 22, 1963, that I called my boyfriend, Kenneth, to tell him that President John F. Kennedy had been shot. Lee Harvey Oswald pulled the trigger on the rifle and America froze in its tracks. Most people I know who were alive then can tell me exactly where they were when they heard the news. I'm no exception. President Kennedy was assassinated while traveling in a motorcade in Dallas. Governor Connally was also wounded but didn't die. Another friend told me he was in school when they announced the news over the public address system.

Maria e-mailed me recently:

> Hi Kirsten, I guess that's a time everyone remembers exactly where they were. I was in

Sociology class (in our junior year, in high school.)
The PA came on and as the Principal said, "May I have your attention please," one guy in class joked, "Due to snow, you can all go home early." We were all starting to laugh, since it was a pretty nice day, when the principal continued, "In a motorcade in Dallas today, President Kennedy was shot and killed…." I just remember hearing someone screaming "Oh no, Oh no!" and then I realized it was me. (I'm sure others were crying too.) Then everyone was crying and the bell rang shortly later for us to go to our last class of the day. Everyone moved through the halls so silently. When I got to my last class, English, we all just sat there in a daze, in our own grief. I remember looking up and seeing the teacher, Mr. Jones, in tears. Anyway, I couldn't wait until I saw my friends after school, when we hugged and cried together.
Love, Maria

Compassion

Walking into the weight loss class, I saw a table laden with books on losing weight. One in particular was called, *The End of Overeating: Taking Control of the Insatiable American Appetite* by David A. Kessler. Toward the end of the class the pencil gave us a few pointers from the book.

After the weigh-in everyone was seated; I counted 10 students. It was amazing that how, after a month, only five out of the 10 had lost two pounds or more. I had lost only 1.8 pounds this week, so to my way of thinking, when the pencil asked who lost two pounds or more I raised my hand. To me 1.8 pounds equals two. When I realized my mistake, she said, "Oh, that's okay, that's close enough." I thought it was nice of her to have a little compassion for me.

It is a good sign when we can have compassion and understanding for people around us. When I was talking to a friend at the pool she said:

Tip # 6
"Thin people need tolerance
towards fat people, and
Fat people need patience
dealing with thin people."

God bless her for saying that. It is so true.

Triggers, and who has what triggers, were discussed. The pencil told us that another student has a "carving the turkey trigger." Then she said, "Oh, I guess it is okay, I didn't mention his name." Sensitivity, tolerance and patience are how we can all share and learn from each other. I will share my trigger with you after talking about the "turkey trigger." I can really see the similarities between the two. The man starts to carve the turkey and then he eats one bite after another and can't stop until most of it is gone. I understand this. It is the magnetic pull that some foods have on us.

Tater Tots

One of my problems is pan-fried tater tots. I learned to fry them when I lived in Georgia. Let me tell you that they taste much better fried than baked in the oven. Here is what happens after a meal of hot dogs, tater tots and coleslaw.

In a large griddle sitting on the stove I pour half a bag of tater tots onto a surface covered in olive oil. It gets hot and then it is time to turn them, and I add more oil. I need to turn them again to get them good and brown, and I use a little more oil. In the South they use Crisco or some type of animal fat, whatever they have, and cook them the same way.

It is time to eat; all the food is ready. I dish out two plates of a fair amount of all three foods. When my husband and I are finished, I take the plates out to the kitchen sink and see, out of the corner of my eye, that there are more tater tots left over. So I grab two or three more with my fingers. Now the TV is on and David is watching the news so I join him. Fifteen minutes pass and a commercial comes on. I get up and walk to the kitchen to eat another two or three tots, whatever my fingers can grab. The program *ends and soon I will be in the kitchen washing dishes, but I will go right to the griddle first and eat a few more tots. This goes on all night until the very last one is gone. I truly feel the tater tots have a magnetic grip on me. The only way to release their delicious power is to not buy them and not eat them, even if I see them in someone else's kitchen. I feel when I put myself in this situation, they truly have the power and I don't. I'm working on that. Every day I work on being strong.*

Other members of the class mentioned their triggers. One liked eating cheese, crackers and wine before bedtime. Two women said how going out to eat was a trigger. Each mentioned a different restaurant, which perked up my ears. Old habits die hard. I feel like the tater tot magnet is coming back to haunt me.

When we go on vacation, the teacher warned us to be more "obsessive" in asking the hotel desk clerk where there is a gym or where you can go for a walk. She told us to bring our own breakfast, like instant oatmeal and a piece of fruit. I had already been doing this, but I do appreciate the tips.

There is a mother and son that come to our group. The teacher told the son to exercise more and the mother to watch her calories more. The teacher does not approve of how I have been watching my calories. She doesn't think that I eat enough. I am not sure which pencil wrote this remark in my food journal. A sedentary woman is supposed to eat 1,200 calories and get LOTS of Exercise. I'm lucky, and I mean really lucky, to get in 45 minutes of exercise a day. Everybody, and I mean Every Body, is different. Each person needs to do what is right for them. Why am I in the class? Am I in the class to run a marathon or to lose weight? For me, the answer is to lose weight. So far, I have lost 14 pounds and I am proud of it. My work has been hard, and I think some of the other people in the class will confess that it is also hard work for them.

The teacher described the cocaine-like effects of sugar. Since I have never had cocaine, I don't know how it is, and she most likely hasn't had cocaine either. We can all read how addictive cocaine is. She says, "I give you a hit of sugar and you want more." I can so relate to this. Chocolate is also like that for me. Once, my daughter-in-law, who knows that I am diabetic, stopped me from myself. She saw me eating chocolate after chocolate out of the box of Christmas candy that we had on the dining room table. Here is the part that I haven't discovered yet. The teacher says that the more you make "not eating sugar" a habit, the longer you can stay off it. Instead of eating sugar, she says to just substitute the right things to keep you satisfied. She suggested something like cheese or nuts. Nuts won't work for me, as they have the same quality as tater tots, only they can be eaten even quicker, as there is no frying on the griddle. Cheese has too many calories, and I can't stop at just a bite. My problem is that almost every food out there is a trigger, so I must be very careful.

Make the Correct Quick Decision

One lady in the class said she had lied about not being able to go to a particular restaurant when her friends invited her to go out. The teacher told us that by doing this she could possibly destroy her own creditability. Her friends might think, why is she not going? Or, let's pick another place that she might like better. It is better to be honest and say that you are on a weight loss program.

Florence brought up another situation where I disagreed with the teacher. Her advice and mine differ slightly. The teacher has been thin for many years and I believe she has lost touch with the reality of being a fat person. Ultimately, her answer is the long-range solution, but when you are fat, one of the reasons you are fat is because you have made many split second decisions that helped you get that way. Florence said when she is at the checkout counter and the candy is right before her eyes, she wants it. Just last week after being "good," she bought herself some candy.

I had what I thought was a really good suggestion. Two months ago it was the Christmas season, and the most delicious candy was just a foot away from my face. It is unbelievable how they can place it so high. It was my <u>favorite</u>, not just any chocolate, but my <u>favorite</u>. I knew I had to move, and I asked David to step forward so as I wasn't trapped there. I moved near the credit card machine to get away from the candy. The pencil would not let me give my suggestion. Instead she voiced hers, which was to first, upon entering the store, buy some berries that you can eat right away after you check out. Sometimes the urge is so strong that you need to do something that very second to counteract the attack of the chocolate. Just walking four steps farther can save you, and then you can go home and eat your berries. The teacher finally let me have my say, but I don't think she liked my idea. Florence heard me and maybe my idea will help her at the checkout line.

Another lady said she goes to church benefits and they have delicious sweet novelties there. Everything is homemade, which to me makes it taste Really Good. Before she walks through the church doors, she puts some sugar free gum in her mouth and starts chewing it. I think this is really clever. We all learn from each other; that's what life is about.

The pencil says we have to get over the "weekend mentality," and the "I've been good mentality," to reward ourselves with food. Food is not a reward. We know that, but it is another thing to live it. I have learned that I need to concentrate on what is most important to me and remember why I am in the class.

Tip # 7 –Focus
"So much of my life is spent just focused on driving race cars."
–Jeff Gordon

Jeff is a four-time NASCAR Winston Cup Series champion. Jeff is a WINNER. He is focused with his eye on the prize.

Do everything in your power and then some more, to keep to your meal plan. That's so easy to say and so hard to do. I try to be made of STEEL. Diet experts say lapses are to be expected, but the problem for me is a lapse knocks me off the diet completely. It brings to mind what it must be like to be an alcoholic. If you don't drink for weeks, then something happens, like a serious emotional upset, and you break down and have another drink, then you start drinking again. My mother had stopped smoking, but then, after my father died, someone offered her a cigarette and she started smoking again.

Generic and Exotic Foods

I know food is meant to keep us alive, but for over 60 years it has been associated with fun, parties, and joy, and that adds up to 60 years of bad habits. The teacher says frozen grapes taste pretty good. I think regular grapes taste pretty good. I wonder why she freezes them. I guess it is because she thinks they taste better that way. She also says once you get rid of chocolate, other foods taste better. I have not had chocolate for a month, and other foods do not taste better to me. I do feel lucky now because the memory of chocolate seems to be melting away. Maybe that is what is supposed to happen. I am still learning. The teacher says that none of us are eating enough vegetables and our assignment for next week is to try a new vegetable. I don't even know what to get. I guess I will have to go look in the store.

When David and I went to the grocery store yesterday, I was very much aware of how it holds no fascination for me anymore. I now have a spiral notebook in my kitchen drawer that contains favorite recipes and I can safely only make one, the fat burning soup. All the rest are way too high in calories. That was my old life. The pencil wants us to focus on loving all the fruits and vegetables. She just means to help us.

Honestly, I'm sick of the words "healthy foods." This implies that what I have been eating in the past is "unhealthy." My parents raised me as best they could, and to think that I grew up on "unhealthy" foods is insulting. Besides, when I was a child, eating those "unhealthy" foods I wasn't fat. In my adult life, an overabundance of those unhealthy foods caused my weight to increase.

I tend to label the two types of foods into entirely different categories, which are: Generic and Exotic. For 60 plus years I had the "exotic" and now, to get my weight down and keep it down, I must eat "generic" foods. There is not much excitement in eating these generic foods. The teacher says if you don't like the new plan you won't stick with it, but I don't think that is exactly true. It makes it more difficult to stick with the plan, but it can be done.

I have several bridges in my mouth, evidence of sophisticated dental work. Every night I spend 15 minutes flossing all the regular teeth that are left, and flossing a second time under all the bridges. There are less than a handful of days during the year that I don't do this nightly routine. Do I enjoy it? What do you think? There are some days that I am really tired and just want to relax. Then it becomes a monumental effort to get the floss out of the baggie where I keep it. I know that I will be able to keep my teeth for the longest time if I floss and if I don't, false teeth will be in my near future. One dentist I had many years ago had a plaque in his office that said, "Be true to your teeth, or they will be false to you." I used to chuckle when reading that, but it is so true. I do an activity that is boring and not my favorite thing to do. I do it every day to save my teeth.

I can eat "generic" foods every day; the alternative for not doing it is knee problems and heart problems, not false teeth. It is just as "generic" as brushing our teeth every day. The pencil can preach and preach to persuade us that "healthy foods" taste wonderful, but she can't make me agree with her. She is only in my life for 10 weeks and then I will be on my own and I will continue eating the "generic" foods that I have learned to substitute instead of eating the "exotic" foods that I ate before.

My Charm Bracelet

My life accelerated during my freshman year at the University of Maryland. I had what would be described as a shapely, almost perfect, hourglass figure, with a little larger waistline than the average hourglass. I collected boys like charms on a bracelet. I wasn't conceited, but I knew this bracelet fact for the truth. Other girls commented to me how lucky I was.

After my father died, Frostburg State Teachers College was out of the question. We couldn't afford it, so I used my little beige Volkswagen bug to drive daily to the University of Maryland, College Park Campus. I was seeing how hard it was on my mother with all the expenses. We only had one income now, and life was harder for us. High school was free, college wasn't. The money that I made the prior summer working at the drugstore covered the cost of my clothes and a little toward my textbooks. Also, I didn't feel I was strong enough, or smart enough, to make it through the rest of my life alone. I knew this meant I needed to find a partner. So I decided my hunting grounds would be the University of Maryland.

It was during my first year that my goals were set on finding the right husband. I should have been focused on academic performance, but I wasn't. My high school boyfriend, Kenneth, was going to Virginia Tech in Blacksburg, Virginia. This relationship, over time, turned into my first serious one.

Once, for the football homecoming game, I went down on the train to visit Kenneth. He had found me a place to stay, a room in a lady's house. I remember little about the dance, but I do remember the lady fixing me fried eggs and bacon while she stood under a hood range light. We didn't have one in our house, which is why I noticed the homey glow it gave to a dawn like setting in the kitchen. She said to me, "Honey, I don't know if you have a ring yet, but you will. He thinks the world of you." I never forgot that. It is just a little comment from a stranger. Once the weekend was over, I was back on the train to Maryland. The falling leaves were turning the trees into skeletons, but I was happy.

By the spring, Kenneth and I were drifting apart. He just couldn't stand seeing me be with other boys. After he came home that summer, things between us were never the same. A year later I begged him to come back, but he wouldn't. That ring that was supposed to be mine was never put on my finger.

Then, for some reason, a new phase commenced. I started having a boyfriend in each class. Here was where the food explosion began. Each boyfriend wanted to meet me for lunch. As it was, I had three lunch hours. One was 11:00 a.m. to noon, the next was noon to 1:00 p.m. and the last was 1:00 p.m. to 2:00 p.m. Each lunch lasted only 45 minutes. Then I used the pretext to go to the next class. Actually this was to make sure the coast was clear for the next boy to arrive on the hour. At least I had the where-with-all to only eat one thing at each meal, just one piece of pizza, or one small side salad, or a few fries. This gave me the proper feminine touch of a lady who doesn't eat too much.

Boy #1 (they will be numbered now, as only the significant ones will have names), I met in English class. He was tall and studious. He barely had time to go out, but liked driving me around in his new car. He wanted a friendship, more than a love affair, which was different than the other boys I had met. Ten years later, I was walking by the television and saw a news program and saw him on the screen as a spokesman for the IRS.

Boy #2 was older than the current college age boys. He was putting himself through school. I met him in geography class. He was Jewish and he worshipped everything German about me. [That is my heritage, but I feel 100 percent American, and to this day read American history, not German history.] He didn't see me as being American, I was his German beauty. He used to take me to the Dairy Queen or the new McDonald's after class. We'd always have milkshakes and sometimes fries. This is in addition to my three lunches. Still I was as shapely as ever, eating all the "unhealthy" foods the United States had to offer. I never thought about food the way I do now. Back then it was just something I enjoyed, and it was a social tool for me to advance in my pursuit of Mr. Right.

This relationship lasted on and off for several years, only to finally end after I started dating my husband, David. Boy #2 got so mad he threw a beautiful white negligee, wrapped in a red box, on my doorstep. It had a card stating that it was a wedding gift. He wanted to "duel" it out with David. He told this to my mother at our front door. Of course, my grandfather had a fit when I wrote this to him in East Germany. He said, "He gives you clothes?" Boy #2 knew I was going to get married to David and this was his mad jealous parting gift. He really wanted to be the only one to see me wear it. He had asked me to marry him, and I did my list of pros and cons, but he lacked one very important quality. I did not love him. His behavior was the rage of a man who was mad as hell at me. But I was safe inside the house with Mutti and David, and after he drove away I retrieved the package. Sending it back would have inflamed him even more, so I kept it and used it on my wedding night.

My grades for my first year at college were barely acceptable. In Children's Literature I received an A, but in Meteorology I received a D. I didn't really study for the final exam, as I hadn't read a lot of the chapters in the book. What was the use when I knew I was so far behind that no amount of effort was going to bring me up to a satisfactory grade? I guess I made a lot of good guesses on the multiple-choice questions, which is why I got a D.

Academically, I was heading into a ditch and I knew it, and so did my mother. We decided that I should go to Gardner Business School to obtain secretarial skills to be able to get myself a job. Back in the 1960s a girl could either become a teacher, a secretary or a nurse. My first choice had been to be a teacher.

I loved the secretarial classes, but they were naturally filled with girls, and my available pool of boys had dried up. I enjoyed studying shorthand, and I was one of the best students in this class. Years later I still write shorthand characters in my mind. On lunch breaks, I would eat my bag lunch with some of the girls in the lunchroom. Boys were not buying me lunches at the student union anymore, so I had to fend for myself. As the girls who sat in the lunchroom with me ate their lunch, we all listened to Motown music, happy to be on our lunch hour. I finished school in nine months instead of 12 and got a job with the National Institutes of Health in Bethesda, Maryland. I mostly worked for older men and women. There was a cute guy who worked on another floor who was a doctor. I tried to bump into him, but he never seemed to notice me. I was either too young or he was too engrossed with his work. I even tried to "run into him" in the parking lot after work, but none of it was successful.

Once, during a break at work, one of the older slightly stout men started talking to me, and mentioned to me how I really should get my weight down. I weighed about 130 to 135 pounds then. I remember wearing a wraparound skirt that day and feeling pretty sharp, until he said this unkind remark. I just figured he was an "old" man in his thinking, because the young men that I knew who were close to my age thought I was beautiful. They liked my curves. To this day, I don't know what was wrong with him. His statement was rude and uncalled for.

I Love David

All the boy fish in the sea were swimming around the University of Maryland, so I decided to work part time, two days a week, and go to school Monday, Wednesday and Friday. Most of the classmates that I had started school with were now seniors, including David. He was my really good friend, who was my comfort and support. He loved me despite all my searching around for boys. I met him at the student orientation when we first started school. We met at a lunch table in the Student Union. I was just as new to college as he was. I often wonder if he saw my uncertainty, but it doesn't appear he did.

He was seated at a table, and there was another girl sitting at the same table. As there were four chairs I asked if I could sit down. David said, "Yes." I liked him and at the end of lunch I gave him my phone number. Years later I found out that he was actually more interested in the other girl sitting at the table, until she opened the newspaper and started reading the sports page. Looking back at many events in my life I can see that so much of it is "cause and effect."

David called me mid-September and thus started the greatest relationship I ever had with another human being other than my parents. It was only several years later, when we took a health class together, that he put his hand on top of mine and I realized that he had amorous attentions toward me.

David witnessed my longing to get to know boy #3, who was a poet. His artistic way with words and his correspondingly different approach to life attracted me. He would talk to me, but his real love, who existed only in his imagination, was Maria, my friend from the ninth grade. She didn't feel any attraction to him at all. I knew this as she and I talked about it. He was barking up the wrong tree. Naturally, this never went anywhere for me, not even one date.

In Anthropology Class I met a student teacher and he and I were friends right away. This was a course I was good at. I don't know if he would have liked a dumb girl or not. Maybe he thought I was beautiful. We often went to the "dairy" part of the school, where they offered the horticulture classes, and ate ice cream together. This wasn't just once or twice; it was Monday, Wednesday and Friday to be exact. Maybe he liked me because I was a little older, 20, and not a 17 year old freshman.

This young man, boy #4, introduced me to Bob Dylan music. By that time, folk music had replaced Motown music as my music of choice. He told me he had separated from his wife. For several months I saw him, not knowing that someone else was watching. One

Sunday afternoon in February my mother answered the phone, and an angry woman told her that I had been seeing her husband. My mother was shocked, as I don't ever remember telling her all the details about boy #4 being separated from his wife. Boy #4 lied to me. He was still married, maybe not happily. Who would love being married to her, a woman who sticks a private investigator on her husband? That was the end of seeing #4.

I found out much later that this is when David saw his opportunity and stepped in to save me and pull me closer to him. It worked. He was as good to me as he always was, but when you have been treated in such a disrespectful way, a loving arm feels even warmer. David had qualities I admired. He was smart and a good person, and someone I could live my life with.

We made arrangements for an August wedding at the University Park Church of the Brethren, College Park, Maryland. We originally wanted to be married in July, but the preacher couldn't make that date. August 9, 1968 was the date that we selected. Unfortunately, my best friend Maria couldn't be my maid of honor, as she was getting married August 10. She never saw my wedding and I never saw hers. We are still best friends.

The searching was over for me. David says that he knew as the years went by that I was someone he could live with. Why I had to bounce off the walls first and sample all the boys, I don't know. But truth be told, when we decided to get married, I knew how bad it can get and how good it can get. The bad was erased from my life in that moment. David and I started our future together.

One of the wedding guests told me later that it was a really hot day. I never noticed. I was aware that my knees felt weak as I walked down the aisle when they played "Here Comes the Bride." Joyce was my maid of honor. She and I had become wonderful friends at the University of Maryland, even though we had met at Wheaton High School. Two of David's sisters were bridesmaids. I wanted a rainbow at my wedding, and had it in the different pastel colored rose bouquets that the bridesmaids carried. They matched the color of their dresses. The preacher read the vows I had written for us. "God is love, and the man whose life is lived in love does in fact live in God.... Love does not consist of gazing at each other, but of looking together in the same direction.... Love knows no limit to its endurance, no end to its trust, no fading of its hope; it can out-

last anything. It is in fact, the only thing that can stand when all else has fallen." When I read the words again that I wrote at 21, I am amazed at how true these words fit my life all during these 43 years that have followed. I feel so fortunate.

After the wedding, there was a small reception at my house. We didn't have money for anything fancy, but my mother had some food catered, and we had German potato salad, little sausages as well as Lebkuchen, a caloric favorite of mine for years. Both families and a few friends were there. I don't know about the other people, but I ate and sampled all the wonderful food on the table. We had rich, good tasting food, almost like a Pennsylvania Dutch assortment. David had just started a new job, so we only had the weekend for a honeymoon in Baltimore. Travel was to happen in our life, just at a later date.

Dopamine

At the first and second weight loss classes, the teacher kept talking about dopamine. This was the first time I had ever heard this word. Like I said before, "These pencils are sharp."

Researching it on the web, I found a definition that is the most understandable. This is by Kristalyn Salters-Pedneault, PhD, About.com Guide:

"Dopamine is a neurotransmitter (or chemical in the brain) that either increases or reduces the activity of neurons (nerve cells). Dopamine has a variety of influences on brain function, including playing a role in regulating attention, cognition, movement, pleasure and hormonal processes. Parkinson's disease, attention deficit disorder and schizophrenia all involve abnormalities in the dopamine system. ...."

Make note of the word pleasure. The way I understand it, whenever certain people (maybe all of us) see or think about delicious foods that are loaded with sugar, fat or salt, our brain gets excited. Because of the dopamine we really want to eat these foods. So you say, "It is not my fault, it is the fault of the dopamine." Your brain tells you that you want to eat the delicious chocolate cake or that you want to eat tater tots. But you know the tater tots don't just sit there–you won't stop eating until each and every one is in your stomach and you have to stop. This is your pleasure going out of control.

The teacher tells us that just the sight of these delicious foods causes our dopamine to go into action. Some scientists think this is like the effect of being a drug addict. Only it is not illegal drugs, but it is food.

Research taken from: Web MD, "Break Your Food Addictions."

Neal Barnard, MD said, "What other term would you use for a woman who gets into her car at 11:30 at night and drives six miles to the 7-Eleven to get a chocolate bar, and does it every night?" She is aware that she is gaining weight, but just can't stop doing this. This behavior is called an addiction. Was the dopamine making her do this? I don't know. I guess the obesity specialists do.

Going Out To Eat

We went to a fast food restaurant that we both liked. I looked in my notes from class and saw that "junk food" is given a bad rap. And perhaps real "junk food" fits in this category. Recently the mood of the country has turned the tide and is "pro health" now. Even fast food places offer "healthy foods."

On foods, as well as cigarettes, the mood of the country has changed. When my mother was young, throughout WWII, and during the 50s, smoking was fashionable, even sexy. Now the government has put high taxes on cigarettes to discourage smoking and has recently spoken out against "unhealthy" eating.

My guess is that in 20 or 30 years the incidence of obesity will decline. Where it will be most notable is on the pre-school and grade school youth of today who, by the time they are 30 years old, will have resolved the problem and be thinner for it.

When David suggested we go out, after six hours of writing and researching this book, I jumped at it. He knows that there are only a few places where I have researched the menus, so we went to one of my favorites. I bought the half-chicken salad. There is no waste and it is the right size for me. As I picked a table where we could sit, I created this next tip.

Tip # 8
Eat small at a big table.

I found the largest round table, big enough for six people, not just the two of us. The restaurant wasn't crowded, so I decided this was where we should sit. It made me feel good. There was still something big in my life that was related to food, but not the food itself. It made me feel big and strong. You might say, "What is the big deal? It is only the size of the table." There is so much more to this than the dimension of the table. It made me FEEL GOOD! Losing weight requires a hard backbone-made-of-steel approach. It is a lot of work. Anything that gives me a smile or lifts my spirits, even though it may be silly, is all right with me.

South Bend, Indiana

The Peace Corps was "in" and Vietnam was "on." Not one friend of mine was for the war. Countless numbers of America's young men had died, and for what? David and I went into a church organization that was like the Peace Corps. We both wanted to contribute to help America. It was a much better deal than just one person giving their life to America. As the bus pulled into South Bend, Indiana, it was four degrees outside, and the wind hit us hard as we stepped off the bus. David was assigned to be a driver and manage a Goodwill-type clothing store to help the poor people in the slums. I was to teach, or rather assist the teacher, at a Head Start program, which was held at a local church. Things were working well until at some point people's attitudes changed. Instead of valuing our work highly, we were thought of in just the opposite way. The group of people we worked for were conservative, Bible belt types, who felt that all men should go to war, so "What were we doing here anyway?" The lead teacher resented that the children liked me so much, so I was assigned to do "toilet duty," which was to help the four year olds go to the bathroom.

The pay for our volunteer work was very poor. My mother sent us care packages of ham, chocolate and toothpaste. The reality was, as one little black boy told me when we went to visit his family, "You are poor." Maybe he knew because I told him we didn't get a lot of money doing this job.

The situation with our "religious" employers grew very uncomfortable. On the day I called my friend that I had met through 4-H, and told her that I had been "fired," she thought a bullet had gone through me. Actually, I had been discharged from my volunteer job. It was at our house that they all met to tell me this news. After that, they stood in a circle while they prayed. I watched them in utter disbelief. Life goes on; we took a few thousand dollars out of our bank account and bought a Volkswagen bug. We drove away from South Bend, Indiana with two suitcases, after a week of fire bombings of cars on the street.

David then had to report to the military, but first he had to take a physical. He was disqualified because of an ulcer. The stress of working in South Bend for a Christian group of people, who didn't act in a very "Christian" way, had contributed to his ulcer. Friends joked, and said I was the problem that caused the ulcer. I am sure that both of us being upset in South Bend made him sick. At the end of the day, I was happy that he was disqualified and wouldn't be going in the Army.

A new phase of our married life started when we were living in Bethesda, Maryland. Our apartment was $120 a month. It was here that a friend in the apartment upstairs taught me how to cook a turkey. She told me not to be afraid of it because of the size, and showed me how easy it was. This was my first step to large family Thanksgiving meals that I prepared later on in my life.

All was well with me. I looked just as beautiful and shapely as before, despite still eating "incorrect" foods. I still ate chocolate whenever I wanted. We often ate canned vegetables and fruit, which are considered not as nutritionally good for you by health gurus. We never had a scale. I was 133 pounds when I got married and years went by and I never needed larger clothes. Weight had not yet started to become an issue in my life, as it is now.

My Angel Baby

At 25 I was pregnant with our first child. Then one day, one month before the scheduled birth, and two months after the baby shower my co-workers had held for me, I felt a large hard mass in my stomach. I thought it was the baby's head. I really didn't know that much about pregnancy. When the hardness repeated a few times in the next few days I thought I had better call the doctor. The baby had not been moving that much, so I just thought the baby was not "active," but still thought my baby was okay. At the doctor's office, he asked me, "When was the last time you felt the baby move?" I said I really couldn't remember and told him about the feeling of the baby's head. He examined me, and after trying over and over with his stethoscope, he could not find the baby's heartbeat. He told me the baby had died. The bottom of my world dropped out.

This next mountain stood before me. He explained that what I thought was the baby's head was not its head at all, but the beginning of contractions, and to go home and wait. At the first sign of labor actually beginning, I needed to come to the hospital to get on with the delivery. I cried and cried, as I knew my baby had died inside me and going to the hospital meant coming home with no baby. The nursery had been set up in yellow, and I went home and closed that bedroom door.

I have no idea how I handled this stress. It wasn't with food, as I can't remember eating very much at all. I was in so much pain that all I could feel was David's love. All I could hear was the voice of my mother when I called her on the phone at work, because I felt I could not get through the next five minutes. Really, that sounds like an exaggeration, but it wasn't. The plan devised by someone, probably David, was to buy me some white paint to paint the back steps, which led from the kitchen to the backyard. I painted, and painted, and painted and painted for about three weeks. Those steps ended up with more than two coats of paint.

Then one day walking down the steps from upstairs I lost about a half cup of blood. We called the doctor and drove to the hospital. My labor was induced, and I woke up in the hospital to be told that my baby girl was in an unmarked grave at a cemetery I never heard of. I loved her. She was my Saint Patrick's Day angel, as I remember her moving on that day. David was strong for me, but both of us were very, very sad.

The doctor said that we could try again for another baby after four weeks and we did. Unfortunately, when the fetus was about six weeks old, I saw a little white covered fetus in the toilet after I had urinated. There was no putting the baby back in at that point. Sadness struck again, and not only that, so did fear. Now I was afraid to get pregnant too soon, and we waited two years. The medical diagnosis of the first baby girl was that I had given birth to an "emaciated female," and the cause of death was "interference of the blood supply."

Still I was young, pretty and not overweight. I was probably 135 pounds now. We didn't have a scale, but it didn't matter because all my pre-pregnancy clothes fit and life went on. Sadness was eventually replaced by daily living. I worked part time now, as I wanted to get myself in perfect shape for whenever I was brave enough to get pregnant again. I prayed to have another chance at a healthy baby and I ate all the right foods. I blamed myself for the bag of *groceries I had carried into the house, before I got the "stillborn baby" news from the doctor. Back then, the focus was on proper nutrition, and exercise wasn't in the mix for the recipe to be a healthy strong candidate to give birth. I eliminated chocolate, and started eating more fruits and vegetables, and ate more protein. Maybe, I was responsible for causing my baby's death. Mind you, I didn't eat recklessly, but my diet was not a perfect pregnancy diet, and did not include additional vitamins and supplements. I prayed and ate right for two years to let my body heal before we started again to try to get pregnant.*

Eat Lots of Fruits and Vegetables

On two of my food logs that have been returned to me the teacher says I am supposed to be eating 1,200 calories a day. The only thing I can say about this magic number is that I don't believe one number fits all. She suspects that I have been eating less, and she is probably correct. What she doesn't consider is that other people in the class can eat two brownies during the week and still lose three and a half pounds. I go lightly on the food, and on Tuesday, our weigh-in day, I do a half fast before class. With all my efforts, including <u>no</u> brownies, I can only lose one and a half pounds. After the teachers criticized people in the weight loss class about their eating habits, I chose not to put myself up for fodder in front of the class. So as I write this book of factual information, my husband refers to my current food log as "fiction."

The truth is that last week, and the week before, and the week before that, I ate the same food. I had a pleasant surprise when I checked my home scale before I left the house. I had lost three more pounds. One week it was only one and a half pounds and this morning it was three pounds.

The teacher told us to retrain our palate to like more fruits and vegetables, and not food like bacon. She explained that if you eat a second apple, which is 75 calories, another 75 calories is not as dangerous as if you eat a second slice of bacon. Doubling up on carrots has less caloric impact than doubling up on pizza.

An amazing comment came from a student who said she is afraid of running into the teacher at Trader Joes, and having sweet treats in her cart for the teacher to see. It was an unusual comment I thought. This is a strategy she uses to keep herself in line.

Salt and Windex

In the class we discussed willpower, and how we need to do extra planning for situations such as when we don't get enough sleep. Just cancel going out to eat that day to remove the extra stress. The students in the class gave their suggestions for handling food that they didn't want to eat. One person said that she sprays Windex on it. Another person said that she sprinkles salt on a piece of cake. The teacher told us to play the tape forward before we eat that cookie. For one minute we will enjoy it, and then all the minutes afterwards we will regret it.

This was the best weight loss class so far. The teachers poked more fun at themselves rather than pointing the finger at someone in class. One of them said that you should forgive yourself for temporary setbacks, but at the next meal, get right back to your plan.

Twenty minutes before class was over we all had to pull a task out of a large bowl. Each task said something that we were supposed to work on for next week. Mine was to limit my snacks to plant food. The teacher told us that there are "no cookie trees." We all laughed. Another lady pulled out her task that read, "Don't eat anything your grandmother would not recognize as food." One teacher told us to remember to eat our colors; she was talking about the different colors of vegetables. Then the other teacher said, "I remember to drink my beer out of a green glass." The class roared with laughter. This was such a fantastic session.

Talk Radio and More

The media plays a role in how we see ourselves. Often in newspapers, on the web and in women's magazines, there are articles about weight issues. Women's magazines have articles about how Lady X lost 60 pounds. There is a before photo in a sweatshirt where she has missed putting some of her hair in her ponytail, and there is the after photo where she is smiling, wearing a cocktail dress, and has her hair professionally done. The most spectacular articles are those of people who have lost 100 pounds. An average person must think, "Wow, how is that possible?" This article draws in the readers. They say to have this kind of success people change their old eating habits and substitute regular exercise workouts. One point needs to be made here: People who eat to excess have that "excess" mentality. This can lead to "orthorexia," where healthy eating becomes unhealthy and normal exercise becomes excessive. This happens to some people, especially teenagers, causing serious malnutrition. It can cause some women to stop their menstrual cycles and cause their nails to fall out. Once I heard someone boast that they did 500 squats. That is not normal, at least to me.

Why do women get such poor body images? Every woman's magazine either has some thin curvy woman on the cover or features an overweight celebrity whose story on how she is losing weight is inside.

I read about a woman who gets up at 5:00 a.m. to work out on her treadmill. She does this for an hour before breakfast, before getting on the subway to go to work. A man swims six or seven days a week and gets on his bike to ride 40 or 50 miles on the weekend. Then there are the young athletes who run track – they run and run, as there is no end to a circular track and their quest for perfection. This is called, "obligatory" exercise, where you just can't stop. This is an addiction, similar to the problem where you just can't stop eating. Both are disorders. Exercise takes over your life instead of food.

There is a television show called "The Biggest Loser." Many people like this show; it's very popular. But to me it seems like a freak show. Where is the sister show, "The Biggest Gainer," featuring the skinny people?

On the radio I listened to a program called "Health Dialogues" on KQED. They discussed the case of a 16 year old girl that had anorexia nervosa. She never thought she was thin enough. When this condition becomes compulsive behavior it can get dangerous. The same is true with overeating; it can get dangerous. Bulimia is another condition where you starve yourself, then overeat, and then purge by vomiting or using laxatives.

Thank goodness I have never done that. I just got fatter and fatter after each diet. Like a friend once told me, each year she just gained one or two pounds but it doesn't stop. I actually wonder how she keeps it so low. I gained 20 pounds during my year in Georgia.

The doctors on the program agreed that the Internet has led to more disordered eating. Young people turn to the Internet to look for ways to lose weight. There is a site called, "pro-ana" where waif girls can go to look at photos of super skinny women and get tips on how to get thinner. This is because thin is in and fat is not.

Another overeating disaster, which happens a lot in adults, is "binge eating." This is often due to stress and lack of ability to handle the situation. That is when a person eats a whole gallon of ice cream, followed by bread and butter to wash away the sweet taste of the ice cream. This can lead to terrific weight gain. Luckily, I have never done this, as I can gain enough weight on my own without this problem.

Many of these overeating disorders are not covered by insurance, which makes treatment by the professionals expensive. Just a routine visit to my doctor is $185 – the "specialist" costs a lot more.

Often there are people that are overweight but don't see themselves that way. I only look at my face in the mirror. I only have my husband take photos of me from the chest up. I'm still pretty, just a little overweight, as I see it. But, a body mass index of 50 is terrible. Before the body mass index, all the doctors did was have you stand on the scale and take your weight. The program mentioned that certain ethnic groups, like African Americans and Latinos, prize overweight women. They say the men in these groups like their women to "have a little meat on them."

The Health Dialogues program then shifted over to Elizabeth Scott and Ramses Munoz. My favorite is Elizabeth Scott, a lady I would love to meet someday. I have so much respect for her and what she had to say. She has an organization called "Body Positive." She tells young girls to focus on their purpose in life and not what they look like in the mirror. She says focus on your beauty. Focus on self-love!

Tip # 9
At the end of your weight loss journey, be happy and love yourself.

This is exactly what I am planning to do. Elizabeth Scott's words felt so good to my ears. I'll never be Twiggy, and I'll never end up like the pencil teachers, but I will give my best; and if, despite all my efforts, my weight stays the same for six months to a year, I'll accept that as where God wants me to be.

Praying For a Baby

After my stillbirth and miscarriage, I worked part time in a private firm. Previously, I was a senior secretary at my Government job, but they knew I was pregnant and figured that I would quit, so the lady who was working under me was given a promotion to take my job. I excused myself and went to the ladies room to cry. She came and comforted me. Since we were friends she came to see me. She didn't think it was right for me to be treated that way. I was told that the reason I didn't get the promotion was because I was pregnant. They don't do that anymore because it is called employer discrimination.

My new part-time job went well. The next two years I prayed like I have never prayed in my life. I asked God to please give me a baby. I knew that I must do everything in my power to make my baby healthy. After I lost my stillborn the doctor gave me a glucose tolerance test because he thought I might be diabetic.

Two years later, before I tried to get pregnant, my new doctor had me take that same test. I was a little afraid, because the first time I took the glucose tolerance test after fasting overnight, at the end of the test I asked David to tell me where the vending machine was. I RAN to the vending machine and I inhaled cookies and a candy bar in seconds. All of this was to recover from the glucose tolerance test. So my fearful anticipation was up, but I wanted to have another baby, so I went through the test. Amazingly, after that second test I walked out of the examination room just as I had walked in. I didn't need to go to the vending machine. This is when I saw that it really makes a difference if you put healthy food in your body. I haven't told the teacher how my diabetic fasting number is around 110. That is not just good, it is excellent for me.

Tip # 10
Treat your body well with good nutrition and all your lab numbers will improve greatly.

Living From Kick to Kick

Two years had passed since my last miscarriage and I became bolder: David and I agreed to try again to have a baby. Driving on Rock Creek Parkway in mid-February I could feel that a baby was soon to be conceived. I stopped working at my part-time job as soon as the good news was confirmed. I followed a "healthy" diet that was prescribed for me and lived from kick to kick of the baby inside me. Once the baby kicked so hard my friend looked at my stomach in amazement and asked if that was the baby kicking.

A month later something scary happened. My baby stopped moving in August, the same month that I lost my stillborn baby girl. I became very upset and sort of froze in place. What was going to happen to me now? Then I told myself, "Heck, I guess it doesn't matter anymore," and I ate a chocolate candy bar. After the last few bites, the baby started moving again. Oh, what joy! What had happened is that I became tense during that month of August because of my experience with my first stillborn baby. It wasn't the chocolate after all. For a brief moment I let my fear go. I have often used food, one way or the other, as a release from stress. This singular chocolate episode was no different. My baby was moving again and I was happy.

During the last month of pregnancy my doctor had me collect all my urine every day, and at the end of the day take it to the hospital to be tested. In case any problem arose, he told me he would take the baby early. I went two weeks longer than my due date and then I was admitted in the hospital. Six times they took what looked like a knitting needle and stuck it up me to induce my labor. I lay there as the sun set, and I stayed there as the sunlight of the morning filtered through the room. Every hour or so someone came to check on me and gave me ice chips, but no food. Actually, I wasn't even thinking about food.

After 24 hours the doctor decided to do a Cesarean section, as my labor never seemed *to progress. I think the memory of my stillborn inhibited my contractions. I was afraid, not of the labor, but of having another stillborn baby. It seems like I could never shake that fear. All I could think about after 24 hours was to get the baby out of me. I was a beached whale and could not have even gotten off the bed on my own.*

Within an hour, my little baby boy was born. I didn't see him at the time, but the doctor told me that he came out screaming. Three years later, before going to the hospital to give birth to my daughter, I asked my son, "Do you remember anything about being born?" He said he did; he told me about the very bright light that he saw. Of course, this was the extremely large round light above my body. It was the last thing I saw before fading out.

Watergate

When my son was seven months old I can remember feeding him in the rocking chair while watching television. The news of Watergate flooded the channels. There were many Congressional hearings in regards to Watergate. This episode started when some burglars broke into the Democratic Party's National Committee office on June 17, 1972. The final blow to President

Nixon came when the Supreme Court ordered him to release more of the White House tapes. The White House was behind a gigantic cover up, and this ultimately forced President Nixon to resign. The next president, Gerald Ford, pardoned Nixon. It was during these televised court cases that I sat feeding my son. I couldn't begin to share the details with you, as I didn't listen closely, but that was what was on TV at the time.

Sunshine in San Diego

When my son was nine months old we moved to San Diego, California, where he took his first steps on the boardwalk. We stayed at a place called Blue Sea Cottages, which doesn't exist anymore. One night, after the power had gone out, I stepped outside to see the total darkness. My neighbor from an adjoining cottage asked me if I wanted to share her marijuana with her. I'm not crazy; I had a little boy to take care of. Why would I accept such a token of friendship when I barely knew her?

A week later we started to search for an apartment, only to find the ones that accepted children were not very nice. They had a small play area in the back, where your children could play. Actually it looked like an area where you would keep a dog.

Life was different in 1974. Now it's illegal to discriminate against children in a rental. We wanted to have a nice place for our family to live, so we decided since we hadn't sold our house in Maryland that we would scrape together every cent we had and buy another home. We wouldn't have to eat beans and rice, but we weren't exactly sure we could make it. Soon, we managed to buy a house.

After that my mother moved to San Diego, and she would come visit us sometimes. She loved her grandchildren, but really did not want to do any babysitting.

I met another mother at a neighborhood park and we became good friends. The two of us formed a babysitting co-op that eventually grew to about 25 mothers. Mostly I watched her two boys and she watched my two children. I stored up babysitting points as she gave tennis lessons. Once I had enough points, she agreed to watch my children for several days, while David and I went to Mexico City. I don't remember what we ate there, but I do know that we drank a lot of Cokes to avoid drinking the water.

My Thanksgiving Baby

It was in February 1976, when I was driving down Genesee Avenue in San Diego, that I had that wonderful feeling in my body that another baby would be coming in nine months. Maybe it is hormones, but that surge of wellness and motherhood sure pounded through my veins.

My daughter was born in the morning during a routine C-section. I was a little apprehensive, but not as bad as I was before my son's birth. I still lived from kick to kick. That is the only way I know to get through a pregnancy. When I was in the hospital holding her, a nurse came in and asked, "Mrs. Crabill, for dinner would you like some turkey?" My daughter is my special little "Thanksgiving Baby." When I brought her home my son looked after her, and on a walk to McDonald's to celebrate "our" new baby, he made sure she was covered with a blanket.

That summer, while I was climbing a ladder to pick plums to make jam, I fell. A next-door neighbor girl, who was in junior high school, lived at our house all day during the summer and lifted my daughter in and out of her crib. She also helped me in any way that I needed help around the house. She never wanted any money, but she did want one gift. It was such a small thing on my part, but I must tell you that she was really happy when she received the Saturday Night Fever record that she had asked for.

The Invisible Mountain

One really bad thing happened in San Diego. The father of one of the girls who played with my son was a Boy Scout leader. My son, and the girl from that family, wanted to go over and play at her house. I went over and met the parents and saw their house, but not their garage. I left, feeling it was okay for my son to go over there and play. But after he returned, he never wanted to go back, and I respected that. So, as before, all the children came over to my house. Months later I found out the Boy Scout leader had been arrested for child pornography and taken to jail. There was one area the Boy Scout leader and his wife didn't take me, and that was in the garage where both of them were involved in taking pornographic photos with young boys. That is the reason my four year old son never wanted to go back. I think he didn't exactly remember what went on, but he knew that things were different *over there and his parents didn't live that way.*

Moving To Maryland

After living five years in San Diego, another job opportunity arose, and we moved back to Maryland. I made a good friend there. We were both social outcasts, because we sent our children to public school, while most people sent their children to a local parochial school. My friend and I worked sorting through clothes at a local Methodist church when our children were in school. The mortgage payment was high for us. The lady in charge felt sorry for me and she told me if there was anything I wanted I could have it.

We lived here two years, and the fancy house that I had in the fancy neighborhood wasn't worth it. Each week before I went to the grocery store I knew I only had money to buy one extra thing. Would it be vitamins or panty hose? Once, which really hurt me, my son asked me after seeing the neighbor's Christmas presents, if we were poor. I said no. We went out and bought a little goldfish, which we named Piggy, as he ate so much.

I remember what a fun time we had when the three of us walked to the school and gathered mulberries from a tree. We were excited about making a pie and eating it at supper. When you don't have extra money that can be a really fun outing.

An upsetting thing happened shortly after we arrived in Maryland. I came down with a bad flu and ear-infection. Not knowing where to go, I remembered some medical offices just at the entrance of the subdivision where we lived. I was a walk-in patient and had to wait. I understood this procedure, but there is one thing that I didn't understand. By the time I finally got to see the doctor, and had been waiting in the cold room with just a paper vest on, the first thing he said to me was: "HAVE YOU ALWAYS BEEN THIS OVERWEIGHT?" I just nodded my head and finally left with a prescription for my ear infection. I never went back. I can't remember what the scale said, as I was too sick to care. I found a new doctor.

Doctors

This leads me to my next topic: Doctors and Weight. Every doctor I have been to in my entire adult life has brought up my weight. Not a single one has offered me any suggestions to help me lose weight. Even my current doctor politely said to me, "If you were to lose a considerable amount of weight, you'd have fewer pills to take." I know he is right, just as I know that I am overweight, but I don't need a doctor telling me that. Do they think I don't know? Physicians should not be patronizing toward their patients. Lectures, nagging and insults are something that patients don't deserve. Overweight patients are becoming the whipping boy of doctors, especially if they can't fault them for smoking.

Our government subsidizes corn syrup, meat and cheese, and not fresh vegetables. Fancy that. Now, I am not trying to totally put the blame on others, but there really was no help for me, only criticism. I have often wondered when skinny people come in with an ear infection, if the doctor asks them, "Have you always been this thin?" What is the point of shaming us?

Any problem we might have is because we are overweight, not because we have fibromyalgia or any other disease. To them, all our problems stem from the fact that we are overweight. With enough brow beating a person can become depressed, and when this happens, they neglect to properly care for themselves. Then they can possibly gain more weight. I read a crude comment on the web. Basically it addressed overweight people as "fatsos," and said,

"Everyone is so sensitive." I strongly dislike any comments that are negative in regards to a person's religion, ethnicity, race, or size. All of these "funny" remarks, posed as "jokes," I don't think are funny.

I found an article on the web entitled "Should Doctors Lecture Patients About Their Weight?" by Tara Parker-Pope. In it, Doctor Robert Lamberts, from Augusta, Georgia said he doesn't lecture patients, and he tries to sympathize with them. He knows that something as simple as eating less calories isn't easy; it's difficult. Where was this doctor when I needed him? All my life I have never had a doctor like him. Too bad I never met him. Maybe if I had, I would not have had problems with my weight during my adult life.

Nutritionists to the Rescue

After writing about the role of doctors in my life, I got to thinking about the role of nutritionists and their recommendations. I never had the opportunity to discuss my eating habits with a nutritionist. They focus on good eating to prevent illness. Also, when you have a particular disease, such as diabetes, they know the correct foods for you to eat to help improve your condition. Researching reviews on the web, I couldn't find any bad reviews about nutritionists. I guess if there are any dissatisfied people, they don't complain. This is so opposite from reviews on doctors giving overweight people advice. Doctors should be helpful and recommend a good nutritionist for you. In my weight loss class, I am getting good nutritional information that matches well with what I am reading.

In my reading, I have learned that fruits and vegetables include vitamins, minerals, antioxidants and fiber. What an impressive list. Experts suggest that eating cold-water fish like mackerel, herring, rainbow trout, salmon and sardines is beneficial. The only thing that I like on that list is rainbow trout and salmon. So, I take two fish oil capsules a day. The doctors I know focus on prescription drugs and not over the counter supplements, except for the 81 mg aspirin.

Whole grains are important, as they provide fiber and help stabilize blood sugar levels. I'm on my own to figure out my diet, but thanks to the three pencils, I am on my way. A person should consume high fiber foods and drink lots of water. Some experts say to minimize dairy products. The teachers told us to go to 1 percent or skim milk because we don't need the extra fat. A good nutritionist will tell you to limit or eliminate alcohol and caffeine.

For me there is no problem with alcohol, but I LOVE caffeine. Basically I love how I feel after one or two cans of diet coke. I mean I really, really LOVE how I feel.

My friend Maria was fortunate enough to have the services of a nutritionist. The following is an e-mail she wrote me. She said I could share it with my readers.

> Dear Kirsten,
> That's too bad that no one mentioned a nutritionist to you. I would have hoped that you could have worked with one, esp. w/ the diabetes. When I first learned that my cholesterol was so high, my internist had me meet with a nutritionist who came to his office on occasion to help his patients. I only met w/ her once, but got the idea of what to eat or not eat.
> Many years later my cholesterol started to go up again no matter what I tried to do. My doctor again had me meet with a nutritionist who also comes in to see patients in the dr's office. That's when I started working w/ her on a regular basis. She made up an eating pattern for me, and then we would meet once a month, until I got things much better and then I would meet with her every three months. I hope she's not mad that I stopped going after the [grand]kids were born. I'll try to find the sheet she gave me when I first started going to her, and I'll send you a copy. She was really nice and helped me a lot. Basically she emphasized reading labels and eating a basic healthy diet with a lot of fiber, lots of colorful fruits and vegetables, lean protein, etc. I

started eating only whole-wheat pasta, breads with at least three grams of fiber, also brown rice.

I think that helped a lot. I would keep a food diary that I would bring in for her to read. After a while I only had to keep the diary one week a month. She would give me good tips and encouragement that made all the good food sound really tasty, so it would get me back on track. And of course the first thing she did when I came in was to weigh me, but she was always nice, even if I didn't lose that much!

Hope that helps with your request for my experiences. My cholesterol and triglycerides really did go down a lot! Oh and also I started eating a real breakfast which I usually didn't do before -- usually oatmeal or something else with high fiber. And we also started eating more fish! I think that's one thing I need to get back to. We haven't had any fish at all this week.

One more thing - she never had me count calories! but I guess the basic outline of what I should be eating was enough. She also said that it was okay to have some chocolate - like the equivalent of three Hershey kisses. I know this is not well written at all, because just when I think I'm done, I think of something else! I should have made a list.

I did like that she said it was okay to go off the eating plan once a week, and just eat whatever I wanted to. She told me how she loves big breakfasts when she is on vacation w/ omelets, and all the other good and fatty stuff and she would let herself go at times like that. It reminds of Rush Limbaugh getting after Michelle Obama because she and her kids ate ribs on vacation. The key is really moderation -- so you don't feel so deprived that you can't wait to get back to 'normal.' the idea is to make the good habits the norm! Whew! love, Maria

Low Blood Sugar

Sometime around midnight, as David helped me move from the sofa where I had fallen asleep, to go to bed, I stopped and sat at the kitchen table. I asked him to help me and give me a small piece of bread with peanut butter, as I noticed my blood sugar level was dropping. That wasn't enough, so I asked for another piece of bread with a little jelly. My last request was for a teaspoon of peanut butter.

Contrary to what the pencils might say, this was not a "too little to eat problem," but rather an "over medication problem." I caught the blood sugar low before I fell into a severe blood sugar crisis. Dr. David suggested that I reduce the diabetes medication

on the days that I exercise. He is so wise. As I said before, NO DOCTOR HAS EVER HELPED ME! Most are big on criticism, but that is it. I quickly forgot about this episode, only to recall it the next morning when I checked my weight and it was higher than I thought it should be.

I only lost half a pound this week. My comment at the scale was "A little slow down, that's good." If I hadn't eaten that "emergency" low blood sugar food at midnight, I may have lost a whole pound. I don't lose evenly, not exactly half a pound a week when I consume my 1,200 calories every day. My body is just not that programmable. As I write and write, I eat carrot after carrot and I realize that I can't let writing this book do me in, then I say, "Especially, NOT THIS BOOK." The more I lose now, the more I will fight to keep it off. To forfeit a 10 pound loss is bad, but to forfeit a 40 pound loss is terrible.

Motivation

The topic of the following weight loss class was motivation. Thirteen students were present. The teacher said "Don't be too hard on yourself, but if you are too lax, you will not lose weight." She defined "grit" as perseverance and sustained interest in reaching your goal. This is not the same as willpower, which is self-control. You can train yourself to have "grit." This perseverance tends to increase with age. After a while you realize that you can't just give up all the time in your weight loss struggle. When I was young, I gave up many times. I am now Kirsten "Grit" Crabill. I have a pencil to thank for that.

This grit thing means you complete tasks on time in an executive way. The biggest roadblocks are failures, setbacks and plateaus. Boredom also needs to be included in this list. The pencil jokes with us and told us how one day we might wake up and realize that we can't stand eating Captain Crunch anymore, after eating it for a few months. To be successful she says you need a high tolerance for boredom. She told us that we need to exercise, but that she adds music to make her exercise sessions more fun. That is honestly what makes water aerobics so much fun. It's the music. You have to realize that the new lifestyle is for the rest of your life and you have to maintain it. You need to bring order to your life, then order to your meal planning and exercise routine. They say that children do better with order in their lives.

The students discussed the things that motivate them. The list includes seeing the weight go down on the scale, purchasing smaller clothes, and obtaining the goal of being healthier. One lady mentioned that she is motivated to do the Cancer Walk to help others. Another lady said she has only 15 pounds to lose and doesn't know why she is in the class. A third lady said she is motivated by the weight loss of the lady who sits beside her.

The lady that sits next to me does not motivate me. Next class I won't sit next to her. I told the teacher that I worked too hard this last month to let my achievements go to waste. She said I was "Very Motivated." I said, "Exactly." I know there is no magic pill and that I will have to work on weight loss the rest of my life. The problem with food is that it is not like cigarettes, which we can completely give up; we need to eat to live. The pencil said we should say to ourselves, "I would like to be in the gym," instead of "I should be in the gym." She wants us to use positive reinforcement. She told the group, "If you feel like quitting, just raise your hand, and I will stop you."

The teachers are easing up on the personal criticism and now joke to make us laugh. They should have started this way. The last person who spoke that evening asked about what happens when you get "muscle" from all the exercising that you do. The pencil told us cheerfully that our jeans would get tighter in the legs. She was comical as she pointed down to her own jeans and then all of us laughed.

*** * * Movie Stars * * ***

Last night I watched the Oscars to see all the pretty dresses. Today I looked on the web to see them again. After exercising at the gym in the morning and then interviewing a friend, I bought a turkey sandwich. By the time I got home I was ravenous. I ate very little of the bread, but was still hungry, so I had a tablespoon full of peanut butter. I swear I think the exercise is sabotaging me. Eat, eat, eat was all I could think of when I got home. I waited too long to get food. This is not good for a diabetic like me.

After eating I went straight to the computer. On the web I found a beautiful lady wearing a red dress. I don't know who she was, this movie star that was at the Oscars. Even the pregnant movie star Natalie Portman, wearing her purple evening gown, was beautiful. I am sitting here looking at them feeling ever so fat. Not just regular fat, but slob fat. How can they be so beautiful? I have lost 17 pounds but I don't feel it when I look at their photos.

I looked at 37 photos of women. How do they get that slim? Can you believe the next thing that popped up on my screen was an article titled "Late Night Eats?" Why? I guess we are just supposed to look at the slim beauties, and then get on with our real life, eating food, food and more food. On the side of the screen I saw a photo of a delicious glass of apple cider. I think I need to click the "back" button to return to the dresses. The movie stars are all so thin. How do they keep food from destroying them? In my weight loss struggle I need to tell myself the following:

Tip # 11
Struggle, Fight, and Say,
"I will not let food defeat me!"

I have only lost 17 pounds and there is much more to follow, but I will be honest: It is hard work. At times I am weak, but I will not be defeated by food. The tater tot army can go to war with someone else. I want to be healthier and, in the process, more physically beautiful, just like the movie stars. I know I will not be a movie star, but I can sure do better, to be the best I can be.

Nadine

Nadine told me her weight issues started when she was a young girl. She started using saccharin to help her with her "sweet" urges. When she was a junior in high school she lost a lot of weight.

She had some miscarriages before and after her first daughter was born. After her daughter was born she gained 40 or 50 pounds. She couldn't get it off. She tried Weight Watchers and lost a little weight. After her second child, she lost 80 pounds and reached her goal as a lifetime member of Weight Watchers. After this she had two more miscarriages. At age 29 she had a hysterectomy.

The years after her hysterectomy she gained a lot of weight. Later, they removed her gallbladder and she lost weight, but she can't remember how. She has tried all the diets and has been up and down with her weight, but she said she was mostly "up."

When her mother died her youngest brother was only eleven, and every day she went over to look after him. She wasn't eating right. The stress of her mother's death, along with caring for her brother, weakened her.

Her safety net in times of stress was chocolate. She'd even make fudge if she couldn't get out of the house to buy chocolate. She tried sweet pickle slices. She cut them up into small "chocolate" size pieces, but that didn't help. She heard that you should try something salty when you want something sweet, so she tried olives. Nothing worked for her.

In the meantime, her back was really getting bad, as she had stenosis of the spine and her discs were bad. This led to more surgery. When she finally had the gastric bypass that she wanted, she had no follow-up care with a nutritionist. Also, there was not any help from a psychiatrist. For six weeks she had to eat instant mashed potatoes, yogurt and sugar-free Jell-O. Gingerly she introduced baby food. She was told to eat a lot of protein. All the food she ate had to be chewed into tiny bits, almost liquefied; otherwise, a regular piece of food would cause her to vomit. On occasion when she went out to eat with her husband, she would forget to chew well, and would throw up at the table. She said she had lost 150 pounds and later she gained it all back.

Her weakness is still chocolate, which she hides in her bedroom, taping small pieces wrapped in foil inside the lampshade by her bed, as she likes soft chocolate. I feel so much for her because it is SO HARD! I don't have just one trigger that I can identify. I find all food that tastes good is a trigger. That means all food in my old life. I know I can never go back.

Later she had knee replacement surgery, necessitated by her years of being overweight. She also had emergency stomach surgery. They thought it was a bowel obstruction, but it was actually scar tissue from her gallbladder surgery. She has had more things happen to her in 67 years than any person should have. To make her life even more difficult to bear, her whole family is angry with her for having gained the 150 pounds back. They should love her and give her support, and not be angry with her.

From 2005 to 2011, Nadine has moved three times. I can identify with this. Between 2009 and 2011, I moved two times. When you move, often you eat too much; I know, because I have been in that situation.

California, Here We Come

One spring day in March, when I could just see three daffodils popping out from the cold ground, we got information that an employer in San Jose wanted David to come work for them. I was feeling really happy about this, because I wanted to go back to California. The movers came and packed everything, including cereal in a bowl with a spoon still in it. I found this while unpacking.

After living in a motel for 10 days we rented a house in Sunnyvale. We spent our summer there. It started off really strange, as we had only been there a couple of weeks when the medfly problem appeared. Aerial spraying was done at midnight. The next day I kept all the doors and windows closed. This was during the summer, with no air-conditioning. Even though the temperature was not that hot, after a while the house got stagnant. Around 4:00 p.m. I couldn't stand it anymore and I said, "What the heck, I hope we don't all die," under my breath so that the children didn't hear it, and I opened some of the windows.

That was a fun summer for us. There were two Vietnamese boys who lived across the street who sometimes played with my children. There was also a nice Indonesian couple who lived next door. I remember going over to visit the wife mid-morning, and I could smell all the delicious food she was making. It seemed to me she would get up first thing in the morning and start cooking, and the food just cooked all day. She told me she was sad when we left, as she liked us.

The very best part of that summer was that almost every day, I would sit with my children and get excited while watching "The Six Million Dollar Man," on TV. The show was about a former astronaut with bionic body parts who worked for the OSI. The star was Lee Majors. He was so strong, and could get out of any situation because he was "bionic." We didn't really know many people yet and the show was a treat for us to enjoy together.

During the day my children ate popsicles. Regular family meals were prepared each evening. For example, one night we had meatloaf; another night we had spaghetti; and on still another night, we had potato salad and hot dogs. There was usually one vegetable to go along with each meal. The meals were not fancy, just basic food. None of us were overweight, and weight was not an issue then.

Field Elementary School

Once school began, my son started third grade and my daughter started kindergarten. I remember walking to school mid-day to pick up my daughter from kindergarten, and then at three we would walk back and pick up my son. We only had one car that David used for work.

A major school event that I can remember was when my son got the "Best Reader" of the class award when he was in fifth grade. I really cannot remember how many books he read. Maybe it was 75 or 100. I just remember the honor bestowed on him.

It is amazing how all the cute drawings never seem to survive the multiple moves and yet certain memories stand out. My daughter had trouble identifying black from brown. For a long time I worked with her on this until she finally got it. I am wondering if this could be hereditary. Now that I'm 60, I also have difficulty telling the difference between black and brown. In addition, I have difficulty with navy blue. Sewing a hem on black pants is really difficult for me and I must take a chair and move the work right beside the window for extra light. Several years ago I read in a biography of Picasso that every 10 years he had to move to a different flat to paint; each time he moved to a flat that let in more light. So, like mother like daughter, this difficulty with color has been passed along, but is not near as serious as the kindergarten teacher led me to believe.

Interest rates were at 16 percent when we moved to California in 1981. It is hard to believe, but we sold our Maryland house at this interest rate. This gave us money to apply toward our next house and assume a loan, so that we wouldn't get trapped into paying 16 percent. There was another house in Santa Clara that we liked, but the one in San Jose with the assumable loan won out, simply because it was more affordable.

Little did we know when we purchased the house that there would be playmates right across the street. My children had so much fun with Darling, Kitten and Eagle, and I think that was one of the best parts of their childhood. Back then our children could play in the front yard, and float back and forth between the two houses, without parental supervision. Darling was the oldest, and she would help the younger ones by reminding them to always look carefully before crossing the street. She was like another mother.

The Evil Mountain Man

The years, one after another, went by until my daughter was in the fourth grade, when something terrible happened to her. A man in a red pick-up truck drove down our peaceful street and beckoned my daughter over to his truck. He asked her if she wanted to get in. She yelled, "DARLING," and he hit the accelerator. Thankfully my daughter was still standing near the street. She remembered seeing a tattoo on his chest and the hairs on his arms. I found out that he lived just a few blocks away. He was living with a girlfriend and also making advances to her junior high school age daughter.

I called the police, who came to talk to me. They said all they could do was to give him a slap on the wrist and tell him not to do that anymore. Because she didn't get in his truck, the police said they couldn't do anything to him. To involve the police in further action would have been disastrous, as he knew my daughter probably lived very close to where he stopped and tried to pick her up. Who knows what he would have done to avenge our reporting him. It was not worth taking any chance for my daughter's welfare, so we dropped the issue. My daughter suffered nightmares and we often had to be with her at night to comfort her, as she was scared. David and I were wondering what to do after that terrible event.

Summer Vacation in England

Fate stepped in and we spent our summer vacation in Cornwall, England in 1985 for David's work. This trip was to see if we would decide to move our family to England. We lived in an old farm cottage in the country, with fields surrounding us. The place was furnished and equipped with a television. There was a separate small building that had a "snooker" table, which is similar to a pool table. For something to do, we would walk to the small building that had the game table, go in and push the balls around.

About 400 feet from our door, we walked to the edge of a field. There was a gate where we could go see the cows. We stood at the gate where my daughter could pet the cows that came up to us. One day, someone had forgotten to close the gate. As I was making the bed that morning, I glanced up to see something moving outside the window. It was a cow looking in directly at me. That was a first for me, and so far that has never happened again.

Often, when the children were watching "Roland Rat" on TV, I would stand out on the patio and watch the grass dancing in the wind. These moments were beautiful for me. We stayed at the farm house for six weeks, before returning home to San Jose.

As a family we had to make the decision about moving to Cornwall for a year or two. David and I talked and felt that if we were to move the children out of their American schools, the best time would be in grade school or early junior high. Still, I wavered back and forth, knowing that my husband wanted to go, but we must consider the children.

One night I had a dream that helped me decide. In the dream the message was to go, but there would be lots of rain. All of us know that it rains a lot in England, so this is not really what the dream meant. There was a "caution" about my dream, but the message was to GO. In mid-January the movers came and packed our things. We were ready to go.

Cornwall, England

Days before our travel began; we stayed at a very nice motel in Los Gatos, California, which was a treat for the children. They were full of excitement, and the temperature was warm enough so that we could all sunbathe. After the long flight we arrived in London. I remember resting in bed while the hotel called the doctor for me. My eyes were tearing and I was having problems seeing, caused by an eye infection that I had acquired during the journey. My son said he watched the Space Shuttle Challenger disaster, on January 28, 1986. I remember hearing it on television, but I wasn't able to watch it. After a day of recovery, we continued on the rest of our journey. This involved taking a train ride while watching the falling snow as we traveled to the West Country, Exeter, England. From there we had a rental car to get to Bude, Cornwall our final destination.

Colds plagued our first two months in England. It seemed we could not get well. I think the extreme temperature change had this effect on us. I spent most of my days doing housewife duties.

We had a very small washer and dryer as well as a tiny oven that could only hold a 9 X 12 pan. My American cookie sheet was too large to fit. The washing machine held only four pieces of clothing. We rented a television and we had to pay a TV tax. The word was out that if you didn't pay the tax, as they assumed everyone had a television set, they would send the government out to check on you.

Despite doing a lot of research before we moved to England, I found many things different than I had expected. Another American who was there said, "They may look like us; they may talk like us; but they ain't us."

British Schools

Other Americans in our group in England put their children in private schools. These, from what I had studied, were to be Britain's best. Only I found out that the British, not the Americans, wrote the literature I had read, and there is a difference in the way we think. Much later, after I had returned home from England, I read that Winston Churchill was independent and rebellious. For this behavior in school he was punished. I came to learn about these "punishments" first hand, on the backs of my children. No one was beaten, but other techniques were used that I consider unacceptable. My daughter was told to put her nose in the sand in front of her classmates, as the teacher thought she did not do the high jump as well as she could have. Once, my son came home from a long day at school without having eaten any food during the day. Someone in the class had misbehaved in the morning and the punishment was withholding food from the whole class for the full day. He was as white as a sheet and I fed him quickly, and heard his story later.

The school was small, which by American standards one would think that means a lot of individual attention for the students. Because my son is very smart, he was used to help give instruction to other students. The sand incident as well as the food incident persuaded me to change my children over to the State schools, for more humane treatment.

There was no longer a meeting of the minds. The British believe their discipline builds character. I strongly believe in encouragement. One British teacher told me *she couldn't find anything to "fault" my son with. Imagine that. She was looking for things to pull him down. All I ever did was to look for ways to lift my children up. I wonder where all those "put down" British kids are now? Maybe they are looking at America seeing what successful children I have.*

Tea and Weight Watchers

Since I was a foreigner I could socialize with all classes of British people, whether they were rich or poor. We were invited to a tea offered by the richest lady in town, and were also invited to a tea at the house of an unemployed plumber who was on the "dole." One had money and the other had heart.

It was in England that I started to go to Weight Watchers. I was 180 pounds then and fought to get down to 170 pounds, where I stayed for a while.

This brings us to British food. I bought an English cookbook that I liked, but the author has a quote in the beginning chapter that I feel is so incorrect that I just have to print it. It's from Virginia Woolf's "To the Lighthouse:"

> "What passes for cookery in England is an abomination….
> It is putting cabbages in water. It is roasting meat until it is leather.
> It is cutting off the delicious skins of vegetables."
> "In which," said Mr. Bankes, "all the virtue of the vegetable is contained."
> "And the waste," said Mrs. Ramsay.
> "A whole French family could live on what an English cook throws away."
>
> *Great British Cooking: A Well Kept Secret,* Jane Garmey.

I Love Shepherd's Pie and Scones

Obviously, the author doesn't think this quote is correct, otherwise, why would she write the cookbook? I didn't even write the book and I strongly disagree with the quote. Every time I talk about British food I always preface my words by saying, "I know many people like French food the best, but…"

My children used to eat "Toad in the Hole" at school. This is a dish consisting of sausages baked in an egg batter. For lunch, my husband and I would sometimes go to the local pub and get a "Ploughman's Lunch," which is a hard roll with a piece of cheese and some extras on the plate. Sometimes you will get an egg or celery or apple slices. Pub eateries don't include the beer, which is an additional charge. I have always liked the British cucumber sandwiches, and once home in America I made them for friends. Also I like another British favorite, Shepherd's Pie. I told my friend Sunshine about this and now she and her Korean family sometimes eat Shepherd's Pie.

I was honored once when I was invited into a British home and my kind neighbor showed me how to prepare dough for making scones. British food is hearty, and hearty is what I have known from my German heritage. Don't tell either country that. The impression I got was that the British hate the Germans, and the Germans hate the British. I don't hate anyone, and I love both German and British food.

One day in February, something very funny happened. We had trouble getting fresh produce from the market in the winter. Every other day I would walk to the store to buy food for the evening meal. For a whole week there was no lettuce in the store. Then I found some iceberg lettuce, and it was like I saw a pale green diamond. Immediately I put it in my shopping cart and had my groceries home with me by 11:00 a.m. There was going to be salad for our dinner. At 11:05 I ate just a little chunk off the head of the lettuce. At 11:30 I ate another little piece. It really tasted good. At noon, I had a little bit more to add with my weight control diet of tuna fish, to make it more exciting. At 1:00 p.m. I was just lusting for another bite. I hadn't had lettuce for so long. At 1:30 I ate just another nibble. Then at 2:15 I drank some tea, and the lettuce at this point, seemed like a special green candy, excellent to go with tea. At 3:00 I ate just another bite. At 3:30 just a quarter of the original head remained, so the decision at that point was to serve my family canned peas for dinner along with the meatloaf that I was going to make. Then, I felt I must eliminate the rest of the evidence of my gluttony, so I gobbled down the remainder of the lettuce. From the quotes about food that I found on the web, here's a silly one:

"Welcome to the Church of the Holy Cabbage.
Lettuce Pray."
–Author Unknown

On my British weight loss journey I lost 10 pounds, which was a good move for me to prepare for another difficult time that lay before me. Another mountain, that I couldn't see, was coming soon. While I was dieting in England with Weight Watchers, I was cold almost all the time because of the restricted calories. I did stick with the plan, and enjoyed sewing in the side seams of my trousers. That was my reward. During these British diet days the ploughman lunch and the Devon clotted cream served over cake and strawberries were not included in the foods that I ate. I was working hard on losing weight, only to later on in life, gain it all back again.

The Sorrow of Cancer

The Duchess of York, Sara Ferguson, who is now a former member of the British Royal Family, was soon to be married to Prince Andrew, the Duke of York, in Westminster Abbey on July 23, 1986. A little over a month was remaining in the engagement when I got a phone call from my mother. She was sick and suspected cancer. I knew it was serious, and after quick arrangements were made to have my mother-in-law come out and stay with the children, I was on my way to Washington State to be with her. Mutti was proud she survived the hospital attempt to kill her, as she described the battery of tests that were given to her. She was happy to finally be home. She was told she could go through some treatment that would extend her life by three weeks, which she declined. Together, we were at her home while bladder cancer quietly defeated her.

After days of bending over to care for her on the couch, I couldn't stand up straight. She wanted to lie on her sofa, and I wanted to do everything to make her happy. The visiting nurse, who came three times a week, suggested that I get a hospital bed delivered to the house. By this time, Mutti didn't seem to care anymore.

I was told to administer the morphine every four hours with an eyedropper on her tongue. I found myself getting physically closer and closer to her bed as she got weaker and weaker. I combed her hair too often, just to let her know I was there. I cried and cried over her. The doctors and nurses at the hospital told me not to talk to Mutti about the cancer, but I couldn't help it. I wept over her and told her she was the best Mutti in the world. She knew I was suffering and didn't want me to suffer anymore. Her last words were spoken about a week before she died, and she said, "Go to sleep, Bunny, I will try."

I will never forget this for as long as I live. She was the one suffering who tried to help me with my sadness. I think a mother is a mother, literally, until she dies. Those last words were really the beginning of her death. I was on my mountain of sorrow.

I felt so helpless; there was nothing I could do. It took an eternity for her to die. Actually, I felt like we both were dying. Her body was dying, while my soul was dying. I called the funeral home two hours after her death, as I wept over her body for those two hours before I could pull myself together to make the call. They criticized me for waiting so long and told me, "Lady, you shouldn't have this morphine in the house; people can steal it." I thought to myself, "So what." Mutti needed it, and did they think I wasn't going to have it in the house so that I could ease her pain? I cringed when they zipped her up in the black plastic bag and I couldn't see her face anymore. After they left, I went outside in the front yard and screamed. A neighbor came over and said, "Are you okay, Ma'am?" I said, "Yes," as if nothing had happened.

There were two weeks left before the Royal Wedding, as I saw a brief advertisement for the coverage of the event on television. I had the television on for about 15 minutes when I saw this announcement. I turned the television off, as it was about four in the afternoon, and I started to plan to dispose of Mutti's possessions. I am the only daughter, so it was all up to me. Keeping busy all the time with repeated trips to Goodwill kept my mind off my sorrow. Actually, that is a poor way to say it, but the work dulled my mind. I don't even know what I ate. I remember once grabbing some cookies off the top of the refrigerator that I had put there. I ate mindlessly; the work got done, and in two weeks I returned home to England to be with my family.

My 10 pound weight loss that I had when I left England just disappeared. I didn't go back to Weight Watchers. I have since found out that Sarah, the Duchess of York, was called the "Duchess of Pork" because her weight had soared up to 220 pounds. She lost the weight later and became a U.S. spokesperson for Weight Watchers.

Once I was back in England, I didn't watch my weight and ate all the Cornish pasties and Devon clotted cream I liked, thus stretching my stretch pants to the maximum. We were in England for another year and *left in the summer of 1987. The children attended the "State" school that last year.*

Once, when I was down to 170 pounds, David bought me a brown suede coat with a fluffy imitation fur collar. We had seen this in a store in England. When I tried it on it fit and looked good on me, so we bought it. It came back to America with me, but I later gave the coat to my daughter because it no longer fit.

Plus Is Really A Minus

There was a big setback for plus size women in America. I never realized what happened, but I wasn't able to find large sizes anymore. I walked over to the men's department and tried on effeminate shirts. I had my speech rehearsed to tell the salesman should he walk by. I would say to him that my husband was about my size and that is why I was trying on the shirts. I often wonder if the salesmen knew I was lying. My lies helped me keep my dignity. After a while I got used to the buttons being on the opposite side.

What happened was that a fashion model named "Twiggy" appeared on the market. She was a pencil thin waif. Instead of being recognized as "anorexic," she was glamorized and this left plus size women in the dust when shopping for clothes. There just weren't any clothes out there for me. I can't remember ever shopping for pants. I had the ones with elastic waistbands that were made of polyester. They seemed indestructible. I had many in my closet, so if one would really get worn to an unacceptable state, another black, navy, or brown one was waiting for me.

My research tells me Twiggy weighed just 95 pounds. Only recently, I think in the last 10 to 20 years, have plus sizes come back on the market. I used to go to the large size women's catalogs; and then, when mainstream department stores started carrying 1X and 2X sizes, I looked on their racks. I was finally able to come out of the closet literally, as I didn't have to wear men's clothes anymore. For years all I could buy was a shirt, and now I am liberated and can buy a blouse. I think it is about time, as 65 percent of American women are overweight. This doesn't make it right, it is just a fact. It is definitely time that they made clothes for us.

Now I am down from 3X to 2X to 1X. I am walking down Mount Everest. I must be careful not to slip. There may be tricky ice bridges out there for me to navigate, but I must stay on the path, despite any and all obstacles.

"Fatigue Is The Best Pillow." –Benjamin Franklin

At the next weight loss class the teacher discussed sleep and how important it is. She suggested that we should avoid caffeine, nicotine and alcohol in the evening. Of particular interest to me is caffeine, as I have mentioned before that I really like it.

The teacher told us that sleep recharges our muscles and brain, and correspondingly when our sleep is poor, our muscles and brain don't get rejuvenated as they should. She told us that if you exercise a lot this will help you get a good night's sleep. We were told that the average amount of sleep is between six and eight hours. Less than 4 1/2 or more than 9 1/2 means there is something wrong.

There are five stages of sleep. She drew lines on the chalkboard to illustrate the differences. The first stage is when a person is glassy eyed and appears bored. If spoken to they can't hear the conversation because their brain waves won't let them. Next is stage two. Fifty percent of our time sleeping is spent in stage two sleep. Stage three is the first step of deep sleep. Stage four is the second step of deep sleep. Then comes stage five, the REM sleep, which stands for rapid eye movement. This is when we dream. Our muscles become immobile, which is why when I am caught in a scary dream and wake up I am sure that I screamed, but I will ask my husband, and he will say it sounded more like a whimper or a quiet groan. He can tell that something is bothering me. But, I was sure I screamed.

Freud says dreams have meanings, but our teacher says it is just the neurons in our brain, which is a reflection of things that have happened to us during the day. I asked the teacher: when I wake up right after a dream and I can't get back to sleep, why do I feel so depleted of strength and energy. She said it is because I have interrupted my brain healing sleep. Doctors have found that depriving people of their REM sleep by medications helps with depression.

Someone asked about melatonin and the teacher answered, "For some people it works; for others, it doesn't. Sleep medications don't work. They just relax you, but mess up your body rhythms." The teacher told us that should we have a bad night that we should not compensate the next day. She told us not to drink lots of caffeine, or decide to skip the workout in the gym as we were originally going to do. We would get wired on caffeine, not get enough exercise for the day, and then we wouldn't sleep well. The same bad night we had before would happen again. She told us to stay with our regular daily plan to get back on a good night's sleep.

The stress hormone cortisol is activated when you don't get enough sleep, and causes you to eat more. The teacher told us not to put the television in the bedroom as so many of us have thought about doing. The bedroom is to sleep and for sex. Don't lie awake in bed and frustrate yourself if you can't sleep. Grab a book and stand up and read it. You will get tired and bored of standing, thus you will want to go back to bed and lie down. If this doesn't work; do it again. Eventually the teacher says it will work. Her lecture was outstanding, and I learned a lot. She is a sharp pencil.

Why Insomnia?

From the beginning of January I have had trouble sleeping. Not only have there been episodes of insomnia that I can't explain, but I also spent my daylight hours pondering this problem. Mid-December to mid-January I went through a month of insomnia, during which time I had a premonition: if I didn't want to face drastic health issues in my 60s, I better do something about my weight. It was my conscience gnawing at me that kept me awake. For a solid month there were muddled thoughts that floated through my half-asleep mind, not revealing the problem. After a month of distress I decided to take the weight loss class that I currently attend. That was a really good decision.

I decided to research the subject of sleep even further. Was my problem that I had slipped from "middle age" into a new category called "senior?" I learned that a senior's sleep is less restful and they often get tired earlier in the evening, and likewise wake up earlier in the morning. They are prone to take naps during the day. Not all of this applies to me. I don't take naps during the day. I fall asleep at approximately 9:45 p.m. in the middle of one of my favorite comedy shows. I sleep long enough to see the end credits or the beginning of the next show and then I am surprised to see how the characters have changed. That fits the senior pattern of going to sleep early. After I started the weight loss class, I beyan getting up at 4:00 a.m. That fits the senior pattern of waking up early.

Then I started wondering if I was depressed. The web says that depressed people wake up early. At this point, I am grasping at straws trying to find the reason for the depression. Joining the class has really lifted my spirits in giving me hope that I can succeed in my weight loss journey. After I gave up the analyzing, I realized, that there is no way anyone, including myself, could say I was depressed.

One night, about a week ago, I had another episode where I felt weak and needed a little peanut butter to avoid another full-blown sugar low at 2:00 a.m. What I discovered was fantastic. Oh, it is not in the sleep books; it is my own original discovery about myself. That morning, after the midnight *peanut butter, I woke up at 7:00 a.m. to DAYLIGHT, after a month of waking up in the dark. It is such a little thing, but my problem was resolved. My waking at four in the morning was not a senior problem; it was a blood sugar problem. All aspects of my life need to be in balance. This includes my diet, my medicines and my exercise. I can't go to bed hungry, as is often recommended in "weight loss" classes; I need to have something in my stomach when I go to bed. DAYLIGHT, DAYLIGHT, DAYLIGHT, I felt like shouting it from the rooftop of my soul. Now, I know what the problem is. I was trying too hard to limit my calories, and I thought I could cut out the 10:00 p.m. milk. But I found out that milk is a whole lot more beneficial to me than just the 80 calories.*

At The Cliff's Edge

Now that I have been shouting my joy from the rooftops, I'll get back to street level and talk about sleep again. Some doctors think that insomniacs have elevated body temperatures, and that their stress hormones are working in a very active way. Different situations can lead to high stress levels. Being pushed too hard at work can lead to "burnout" levels where all the employees do is work, work and work. The 40 hour work week, which is what they are "being paid for," exists only on paper. One thing can be worse than too much work and that is unemployment. We also have been through this. I will cover my personal experiences later.

Unemployment can affect much more than sleep, it can also impact eating. The following is from the *Insomniac* book I was reading. It is from a physician in Alabama at a free clinic:

"Most of my patients cried yesterday. This happens pretty regularly, but not most in a few hours. Goodyear is buying Dupont and closing the plant here; a woman, who's worked there for 24 years, knows nothing else. A woman, who has worked for a nursery since she was 19, is being laid off. People aren't buying shrubs." *Insomniac,* Gayle Greene, Page 155.

Drastic changes with eating food can occur with this stress. Some people will eat less, some will eat more, and some will run to their comfort foods. Here's another example of a stressful situation that can make a person run to food. This is taken from the same book, *Insomniac*, which I quoted previously:

"I went to my doctor, asking for a benzodiazepine because that is the only thing that works for me. He said no, no, they're addictive. He then proceeded to tell me that whenever he has a sleeping problem, he just writes his worries down on a piece of paper and tears the paper up –

'like so,' and he held up a piece of paper and ripped it in two. Like, that's all there is to it. I just stood there, stunned." Page 172

All you have to do is change a few words and say, I went to the doctor asking for help with my weight problem, requesting a diet pill, and he said, "No, no, that could be addictive." He then proceeded to tell me by writing down on a piece of paper to "Just Eat Less Food." Like, that's all there is to it. If you were a smoker, he would write on his prescription pad, "Just Stop Smoking." This advice can lead the patient to eat too much food, or get upset and smoke that next cigarette. Maybe the best answer is to see another doctor, but many people will react in some type of emotional way first. The doctor should not shift the blame to us so quickly, as the least he could do is be a little more compassionate. Sometimes a person will see a doctor for a snoring problem, only to be told that he should lose weight first.

I found one solution to help me with sleeping and eating. It is to take a hot bath before I go to bed. I enjoy how my body feels, as the bath is very relaxing. Afterwards I want to relax in bed and there is no extra strength to walk over to the kitchen to get something to eat. I have found a positive behavior to substitute for a negative one. The only problem is that I can't take a bath every hour.

A Mountain of Food

An addict who has gone to extremes can't perform well at tasks he is assigned. His addiction has blurred his brain. There are drug addicts, sex addicts and food addicts. I now realize that I had a serious food addiction. My symptoms had to be really graphic for me to see it. I was no longer just overeating.

I used to go to potluck lunches and enjoy myself. I noticed that I would eat a little more than the other ladies. Many of them were small, and of course, they would eat less. It was acceptable for me to eat larger portions, as I was larger than they were.

The last potluck demonstrated the truth about my food problem. I finally saw it. I was one of the first to get up and go over to the food table. I put two pieces of pizza on my plate, not just one, which was what I should have done. If I thought the other ladies around me were busy talking, I would put three pieces on my plate. The third one would cover the second one, so that it was not so obvious. I generously helped myself to every dish on the table. I'd already gone back to my seat and started eating before everyone had served herself. I took a napkin to hold the cookies, pizza and all the other dry items that I wanted to take home. I quickly wrapped them up and slipped them into my purse, watching to make sure that the ladies around me were talking so they didn't see me. If I got discovered, I'd say that the food was to take home to my husband. He does get some of it, but the truth is we share it. Then I ate some of the mile high portion of food on my plate, so that my plate looked like the plates of the other ladies that were sitting around me. I'd eat so fast that it felt like a bomb had just exploded in my stomach. No one saw that. My secret was hidden.

Part of my solution is that I can't go to potlucks anymore. My illusion of control is that I didn't go back for second helpings. I am wondering if drug addicts hide the truth from others. I am embarrassed that I have done this. I couldn't stop. I feel bad. I needed to hide my crime by rearranging the food on my plate so it looked lady-like and resembled the other ladies' plates. I will have to work on this the rest of my life. The major obstacle for me is that delicious food is everywhere.

Please Help Me I'm Falling

Bill Withers wrote the song "Lean on Me." It is a show of support to the person who needs help and is not meant to be taken literally. Going back to the weight issue, who really wants a 300 pound person leaning on him? These 300 pound people are usually not out there. They are at home because they feel that no one likes them anyway as they are so large. They are struggling. They feel helpless and ashamed, which is why they stay home. They cannot control their overwhelming urge to eat. Who is treating these overweight people? The wealthy can buy lots of help. The rest of us are not so lucky. The answer as to who is treating us: we have to do it ourselves. The "Buck Stops Here" was a phrase that President Harry S. Truman liked. He kept a sign with that saying on his desk.

What happens to overweight people when they fall through the cracks? When you are 150 pounds the crack is only 15 feet wide and there is a friendly person in a weight loss group to talk to you. When you are 200 pounds the gap is 20 feet wide. You are starting to really look fat to everyone else. Maybe a few people will talk to you, but only if you talk to them first. When you are 300 pounds the gap is 30 feet wide, and you can't socially stick out your arm because it is so fat that you are embarrassed. You are not at the weight loss meeting. You are sitting at home watching a television show behind your crying eyes. The food has a hold on you, just like my tater tot army. Before, they were winning. Now, Victoria told me that when she passes the freezer section in the grocery store, she will sword as many of them as she can to help me.

I took a little test to see if I was a drug addict. 1) Do I have hidden food/drugs in the house? Please focus in on the first word, which is "food," as that is what I am talking about. 2) Do I feel guilty about my behavior when I know I eat more food/drugs than other people? 3) Have I used food/drugs to relax and feel better? 4) Sometimes I can't stop eating food/drugs even if I want to. The answers on the quiz indicated that if I did just one of the things, that meant I had a problem. I marked four of them that I just shared with you. This test came from the article *Drug Abuse and Addiction Signs, Symptoms, and Help for Drug Problems and Substance Abuse,* by Melinda Smith, M.A., and Joanna Saisan, MSW at www.helpguide.org.

Tip # 12
In making a quilt, it is your perseverance and aim for perfection that makes the blanket come out beautiful in the end.

I'll have to keep working and striving for control over the food I eat for the rest of my life, so that the blanket I wear will be beautiful on the outside, the way my heart is on the inside.

As I was walking down the hall with a thin friend to interview her, I told her that when I was young I had many boyfriends and was beautiful. She said, "Kirsten, you are beautiful." Oh, how good that felt. A fat person needs lots of love, and not criticism.

Mountain Of Motherhood Fear

In the summer of 1987 we returned to San Jose. My daughter entered the sixth grade and my son entered the ninth grade. My son was tested to find out which classes they should place him in; I was amazed that he was placed in Algebra Two, never having taken Algebra One. I guess he figured out the basics himself, as he never talked about any math instruction in England. Perhaps it was there, but he never talked about it. For a week after we came back he was referred to as "The boy with the English accent." Then this label disappeared, and so did his accent.

The following school year turned out to be a scary one. My daughter was home sick for about two weeks with what seemed like a nasal/stomach disturbance. It wasn't so bad at first, but then it got worse. Just when I was thinking perhaps she was improving, and was considering that it was time for her to go back to school, she took a turn for the worse. Each day she became sicker until she couldn't get out of bed and was very weak. When it was obvious that she wasn't improving, we took her to the hospital and she was admitted. Her pediatrician thought it was a stomach problem, and appeared to be relaxed about it. I kept asking him to please check everything, as I was worried about her. The doctor diagnosed her condition as depression.

The doctor said that my daughter's problem was "her neurotic mother." I could see that working with this doctor was going nowhere. What mother wouldn't have been upset? I asked the nurses at the desk to help me get another medical opinion. Another doctor stepped in and did a CAT scan on her head to discover that her nasal passages were completely clogged, compacted with mucus. The doctor immediately started an IV drip of antibiotics, and within a few hours a smile returned to my daughter's face. My heart was lifted out of the ditch and I could see the sun shining again. The second doctor told me later that my daughter most likely had only five more hours before she would have died. Please listen to this, dear reader: Please be a little neurotic to save the life of your child. At follow-up visits to the new doctor I twice saw the old doctor in the hall walking toward me, and each time he bowed his head looking at the tiles on the floor so as not to look at me. I really didn't care about him. My daughter was well, and he was the one that had the problem.

My daughter had various summer jobs once she was old enough to convince employers that she was old enough. One of the first jobs was working at a doughnut shop, where she was up at 5:30 a.m. to get ready for work. What was so amusing was that the doughnut shop was next to Weight Watchers. She also worked at a yogurt shop. Then she worked at an ice cream store, where she later bragged, "I was in management, even back then."

When the children weren't in school or working they played at home. "Kick the Can" was a game they enjoyed with the other kids on the street. They worked hard at school and at their jobs. My son worked at an Arcade one summer, and for many summers worked for a neighbor with his electronics business. Both children were busy and happy. I encouraged them in their lives and told them to always feel free to come to me to talk about anything that was bothering them.

"Criticism Comes Easier Than Craftsmanship"
–Zeuxis (Greek Painter ~400 BC)

Never once did I ever focus on weight with my daughter. She was average, just like I was average. I had a good friend, who was very slim, but she was married to a lumberjack of a man, and unfortunately her daughter had a larger build than average. My friend mentioned her concern to me about this subject, and I didn't know what to say to her. I think this problem arises when young, thin mothers (and maybe fat mothers now) just focus on the flaws of their children. I have never done that, and fought like a tiger to pull my children out of a situation where that was happening. It must be hard on a young girl when her mother gives her a displeasing look as she reaches for a second helping at dinner. I think it would be like a slap on the hand. The mother needs to talk to the girl in a loving voice, and not at mealtime, to give her suggestions to reach for the lower calorie foods. Children want their parents' love, not their disdain.

Some mothers even have harsh remarks when they see their daughters eating a piece of birthday cake that they brought home from a party. They will make a snide remark telling their daughters not to blame them when their favorite jeans don't fit. Disapproving looks, and disapproving remarks, are so destructive to a child's ego. It is better to lift them up, go really high, and educate them at the same time. That is what we did for our daughter.

Do You Know How To Walk?

For years my daughter walked in my son's shadow of A and A+ grades. She expressed an interest in going to modeling classes, so my husband went around with her to interview the instructors. Many were focused on just a person's outward appearance, but one stood out in her views. She told my husband that her teaching works from the inside out, which meant that the last thing to be covered would be the clothes. She told my daughter, that when she finished the class, she would be able to dress herself from a Goodwill store and look like a million dollars. She was RIGHT. After the second class my daughter came home and while we were all sitting in the living room, she said to her brother, "Do you know how to walk?" He just sat there, sort of dumbfounded by this question, and shrugged his shoulders with a resigned attitude of "Well, I guess so." He never actually said a word, but we knew this was what he meant. Then my daughter walked across the room to demonstrate the correct way to walk. Little did we know that was the turnaround in her life, where she no longer walked in her brother's shadow. It was the beginning of her ascent toward success.

Struggling To Survive On the Mountain

Once, in 1991, my husband almost lost his job, but was saved during the last hour on a Friday afternoon. His boss had found him a position after David worked all the way to the last hour, thinking it was his last hour of employment. But, in 1993 disaster hit. It was

Christmas 1993, when David and 500 other employees, were given a group "exit interview." It was nothing personal, but it hurt just the same.

I had always stayed at home, as my last job was before my son was born. At first I dressed up and went to an interview at a real estate office. My knowledge in this field meant nothing to them. They advised me to go to a community college and take computer classes, and then come back.

When I was out walking, I saw a Help Wanted sign in the window of a dry cleaner. Again, I made sure that my appearance was neat, and I walked in with a positive attitude. While talking to the owner, I told him that I could learn what I needed to know, and that I was a very reliable worker that he could count on to be at work during my designated hours. He told me to fill out an application. More than a week went by. Two weeks later no one had called me about the dry cleaning job. Then, one afternoon, I got really brave and walked down to the shop. Looking through the large front window I could see a young 17 year old girl standing where I should have been standing. I walked down past the other shops, turned around and walked home. Was it my age? Was it my *weight? What was it? She was cute and young, which is probably why she got the job. Maybe she had prior dry cleaning experience; I'll never know. What were we going to do? I always thought of us as a family, not just myself. Maybe if I had been more selfish, I would have controlled my weight more, and I would have been slimmer, and got the job.*

Our home had four bedrooms, but only three were being used. We decided to paint one and rent out the room. We found a quiet young man to rent a room from us. He stayed with us for a year and a half.

Tragedy in Oklahoma

On April 19, 1995, I was sitting in our family room, on the sofa near the steps, when our renter walked down the steps. At that same moment flashing across the television screen were pictures of the bombing of the Alfred P. Murrah Federal Building in downtown Oklahoma City. This was the worst terrorist attack on American soil prior to September 11. One hundred sixty eight people died, including 19 children under the age of six. I will never forget our renter's words, "Kirsten, I hope my people didn't do this." I told him, "Don't worry, it doesn't make any difference in our relationship with you." I think he felt relief that I felt that way. Minutes later he left to go to work.

Children, Chickens and Charity

During this half year of unemployment, my husband found part-time work. He was just a few dollars over the cut off line so we couldn't get any unemployment benefits. With the $300 a month I received from our renter I could buy groceries for all of us. Many of the grocery stores often had the "Buy one chicken, get the second chicken free," and that is exactly what I did. Our renter would give us a few extra dollars when he would eat with us, but it was not regularly, as he would often eat out. My husband, even today, remembers all of the chickens that we ate.

The wife of the couple who lived across the street said her church gave out gift boxes at Thanksgiving, and asked me if it was okay for her to put our name on the list of recipients. I said we would love to receive a gift box, and thanked her very much. Days later I went over to her church to pick up my box. I never felt ashamed. It was just reality, and we could surely use the help. When I got the box I never looked in it, and went right home. I was home before my children came home from school.

My son helped me unpack the goodies. Six or seven of the fattest oranges came out, followed by really plump celery stalks. Then we lifted out a dozen extra-large eggs, and a nice loaf of bread. This was all quality food. After my son and I examined the loot on the table, he said, "Gee Mom, we should be poor more often." I told him to hush his mouth and not talk like that. Our cost cutting has been visible to him, but no one starved. I never had a part-time job, but that probably would have just brought in the rent money anyway. This is when we realized that the mortgage payment on our "larger house" was really hard on us. Later we sold our house and moved back to the house we had before, the house that had been rented out.

On a cold winter morning in 1996, my husband went back to his old employer to sign his work papers. That afternoon we rode in a limo to the airport. New Jersey would be our home for a few months. The limo ride was fun and luxurious, but what it stood for was even better. We had a full-time job now and that FELT SO GOOD.

Pretty Rare, Beyond Compare Student of the Year

The children were in college now, and no longer required our constant attention. My daughter first went to a community college in San Clemente, California. Her best friend's mother said that four girls could board at her deceased grandmother's house. My daughter also tried to get jobs in Hollywood, and got parts as an "extra" in movies. I saw a commercial she made.

Later, at Seattle Community College, she got her AA degree. She worked part time, where she ran across a most unpleasant co-worker, who bashed her with insults and said she would never go anywhere without a degree. I call her the "witch-bitch." Nobody talks to my daughter that way. After coming home to San Jose, she finished her BA degree in Public Relations.

Before graduating, something spectacular happened. Throughout college she didn't have the low-wage jobs that she had when she was younger. She wrote essays that offered scholarship money. She earned some money this way, which she spent on school clothes. An opportunity arose to try out for "PR Student of the Year." She had to stand in front of the judges and tell them why the Bahamas was an ideal location for them to steer their business.

I remember on the afternoon before we left to fly to New York we were making copies and PowerPoint slides at Kinkos to take on that trip. I was amazed that it cost $180, but I would have paid $300, as this was really important to us.

She was one of the five finalists that were flown to New York. I paid my own way, as did a good college friend of hers. We both were on a late night flight to New York. I can't remember what we ate, just whatever was offered to us. I wasn't even weighing myself at the time, and thus I have no idea what I weighed.

I was not invited to attend the ceremonies, but waited in the hotel room with her friend. We went out once to the street and I ate a large hot dog. I couldn't help it. I wasn't hungry, but I was anxious and nervous like any caring mother would be.

When my daughter arrived at the hotel after her evening festivities, she joked with us saying someone else had won, but I could see by the twinkle in her eyes that she was the WINNER. She won out over 500 students from across the United States. Victory is so sweet!

We celebrated the last two days we were there.

Stanford Graduate School

Parallel to this event my son applied to graduate school. He had graduated summa cum laude from San Jose State University with a degree in electrical engineering and was looking for graduate schools to attend. Just for the challenge, he applied to Stanford University.

Not only was he accepted at Stanford University, but he was offered a teaching assistant position, and thus we didn't have to pay tuition. The staff from the electrical engineering department liked him, and gave him book vouchers, which he used to purchase textbooks. He graduated two years later with his Master's Degree in Electrical Engineering. Several years after that, along with his full time job, he returned the kindness extended to him and taught one evening class at San Jose State University for a few semesters.

Both children soared like eagles, not because I punished them for failure, but because I did the opposite; I praised them for everything that they did right in their life.

When you train a dolphin, you don't hit him with a whip; you reward him with a fish.

"Attitude Is A Little Thing That Makes A Big Difference" –Winston Churchill

When my children were young adults they were active in all aspects of their lives. No one was overweight except me. We all just "lived," and we didn't go to a gym to "exercise" daily, which seems to be the "in" thing to do now. I decided to research exercise, as I know it will be covered in class later, but I want to share my views from a non-athlete's position. I am very upset to see the judgmental way some of the thin world sees the fat world. Some thin people feel that just walking three times a week isn't even real exercise, as it is for wimps who are not physically fit. Serious exercisers love to sweat, and they can walk up and down hills and not get winded like their fat friends.

I heard one comment that made me sad and made me realize the gigantic gulf between "fat think" and "thin think." People working on losing a few extra pounds at my friend's gym commented on how the fat ladies think they are doing real exercise in the water, and then they go out to eat. Fat people don't say things about thin people who exercise to exhaustion and return to the locker room with red faces. What I am trying to point out is that fat people don't criticize thin people. Most of the weight jokes are about fat people, not thin people, who seem to wonder why fat people are so sensitive.

Exercise Equals Energy

There are some really good reasons to exercise. It can help improve your stamina, build your strength and improve your sleep. There are many gentle ways to start with exercise, such as Feldenkrais, Tai chi and Yoga. Lifting weights and working on the machines is for the hard-core exercisers. What I am trying to do is just MOVE! I know this is not good enough for my teacher, but for me, with my difficulties in trying to adjust my diabetes medications, it is a beginning. Who knows, one day I may transform from a square dancer that gets out of breath after just one dance, to become a water aerobics instructor. You are laughing, but this person exists. She is a friend of my best friend Maria. I need to make small life changes in the beginning, and then improve all the time. I like increasing my flexibility, because it gives me more power over my body. Exercise can help some people who are stressed, although, that hasn't worked for me. I run to food first, not to the gym.

I must tell you that for me to talk about exercise is like a penguin telling you what it is like to vacation on the equator. There are plenty of books saying what the professionals think, but I am a beginner in the exercise world, so my views will be different.

"I Love How Exercise Clears My Mind"

People exercise "to stay healthy and live longer with a sense of well-being." That is what Wiki Answers says. Many people don't like to exercise. Often women just give up because the beautiful body they thought they would be getting just isn't there. When there are small children at home, many women put the children's welfare first and don't take time to exercise. That is just what I did. Some people say they don't have time; real exercisers make the time, and get up at four in the morning if that is what it takes. A cashier I spoke to got up at five and did 40 minutes of exercise to "stay trim and fit," because she said, "I love how exercise clears my mind."

A non-exerciser will wonder about this, but a pro understands the quote exactly. I know a lifeguard who does 100 laps in the pool in the early morning. I know a lady whose goal is to do 500 squats. Wow, this is jumping way out of my league. They claim athletic people live longer than couch potatoes. I guess I better get up out of this chair and go take a walk.

Today our society is obsessed with fitness. I can't remember this from before, but I think it is due to all the overweight people in America. I think the bottom line is that exercise needs to be enjoyable or you won't stick with it. When the music stops that I am listening to while doing water exercises, I just stop. The joy just vanished out of the exercising. I'm the true imposter in the gym, but I am trying. At least I am not sitting home eating ice cream as many thin people might believe. What motivates me is the fun and music. There is one thing that intrigues me in my research: it is a statement that says, "One may improve his brainpower by exercising." That really excites me. I'll just put on the rock and roll music at home and dance. Maybe I'll get smarter.

Get Moving To Love Your Heart

Measuring heart rate is a big deal, and very important in exercise circles. There is a Borg scale where numbers are assigned to intensity of the exercise. Six to 11 is very light, warm up, cool down motions. Twelve to 13 is somewhat hard, and 16 is very hard. I have no idea what 16 would be like, as I have never been there. At least this is somewhat understandable and easy to calculate, unlike the next bit of math. For this, you need to be a mathematician. When doing any exercise I can't process these formulas. Maybe if my mind improves with exercise, I'll become a math genius. HR equals heart rate; I understand that. Where I lose it is at the rest of the equation.

Other often cited formulae are:

$HR_{max} = 206.3 - (0.711 \times age)$
(Often attributed to "Londeree and Moeschberger from the University of Missouri")

$HR_{max} = 217 - (0.85 \times age)$
(Often attributed to "Miller et al. from Indiana University")

$HR_{max} = 208 - (0.7 \times age)$

In 2007, researchers at Oakland University analyzed maximum heart rates of 132 individuals recorded yearly over 25 years, and produced a linear equation very similar to the Tanaka formula–$HR_{max} = 206.9 - (0.67 \times age)$–and a nonlinear equation–$HR_{max} = 191.5 - (0.007 \times age^2)$. The linear equation had a confidence interval of ±5–8 bpm and the nonlinear equation had a tighter range of ±2–5 bpm. Also another nonlinear equation was produced – $HR_{max} = 163 + (1.16 \times age) - (0.018 \times age^2)$.

The 2010 research conducted at Northwestern University revised maximum heart rate formula for women. According to Martha Gulati, et al., it is:

$$HR_{max} = 206 - (0.88 \times age)$$

A study from Lund, Sweden gives reference values (obtained during bicycle ergometry) for men:

$$HR_{max} = 203.7 / (1 + exp (0.033X (age - 104.3)))$$

and for women:

$$HR_{max} = 190.2 / (1 + exp (0.0453 x (age - 107.5)))$$

These formulas are courtesy of the Wikipedia article *Heart Rate*. Actually, these formulas confuse my brain. I find these formulas difficult to understand, as math was never an area where I excelled.

There is also the "Zoladz" method, but it is not any easier. To read more about this go to the Web http://en.wikipedia.org/wiki/heart-rate.

There is an easier way. Isn't that great. All you have to do is buy a "target heart rate" monitor. You wear it like a watch. I saw five of them in photos ranging in price from $36 to $62. Now, that's not a bad price, and you'll save a whole lot of calculating.

Only Three Easy Payments of $39.95

The price of the target heart rate monitor seems reasonable compared to the exercise machines that you can purchase. I saw an article put out by a trainer telling the readers to check with a trainer first before becoming a victim of the exercise machine industry. That really does seem like good advice. There are infomercials that promise results in a really short amount of time. Seventy different machines were reviewed. There were treadmills and "ab" machines, "butt" machines, and even machines to help you breathe better. The prices can go from $39.95 to over $1,000. Watch out. Buyers beware.

The Excitement of Exercise

On a much lighter note, I would like to talk about what I saw and felt when I read some sport magazines. From the "Golf Magazine," December 2008, Volume 50, Issue 12, page 73, I read this suggestion:

> "PLAY SMART; Eliminate Big Numbers
> By Controlling Your Misses."

In the "Young Rider" Magazine, a magazine for horse and pony lovers, May/June 2004, page 36, they advertise a vacation in the Canadian Rockies. They say for many it is a "magical and life-changing experience." As I sat in my chair reading this I thought, "Wouldn't it be wonderful if I could ride a horse and be there with them?"

The third magazine I looked at is called "Adventure Cyclist," February 2011. As I looked on the front cover I realized my body type doesn't match that of a cyclist. They are usually tall, thin and have strong legs. Despite that, I secretly wished I could go on the four-day, three-night Mount Hood Loop trip in Oregon. Once, when I was eleven, I went to a lake near there, and while floating in an inner tube I could touch the top of Mount Hood.

Or, I could go on the "Great Ohio Bicycle Adventure." That trip involves 3,000 people, for seven days and nights. I felt like crying as I wish I could be there with them on all the trips. My fat and my inability to ride a horse and a bike are holding me back. As I see it, these vacations show the "Excitement of Exercise." Maybe someday I will be there with them.

A Twenty Pound Loss

The next weight loss class was mostly a review. Eighteen people were there. The comment made to me at the weigh-in was, "You are a model student, your weight loss is consistent and you have structured amounts of food that you eat each day." I had achieved my 20 pound weight loss goal.

Students were complimented on the exercise they did, but the teacher reminded all of us that it is a "weight loss" class, not an exercise class. She said that once we have been in the program for a long time, she wants us to strive for half a pound to a pound of weight loss each week. She was joking with us as she said, "Walking the dog is good for the dog." Walking is good for me. My knees don't hurt when I walk, so for me, gym exercise is not the best. The pool activities are the best.

Success, Struggles and Birthday Parties

The teacher asked us, "What are you having success with, what are your struggles and what are you going to change for next week?"

Florence said it is a constant struggle for her to always be aware of what she is putting in her mouth. The teachers commented on a remark that was made to them which was, "Well, it is easy for you." One of the teachers set us straight and said she has been working hard at it for 28 years and said that she does it because she doesn't want to be obese again. I am not sure what she weighed at her fattest, but she is now probably 110 pounds; let's say she lost 50 pounds, which would have put her at 160 pounds when she started. Many American women would not consider that fat.

We were reminded that there are always going to be birthday parties, as two of the women commented on the difficult week they had because of birthday parties. When it came my turn to answer the three questions, I said that I had been successful when I added in the glass of milk before bedtime, which helps my blood sugar level at night. I also said that I would like to increase my exercise a little. The last question of the three was, "What are you going to change for next week?" I said that I didn't plan to change anything. The teacher said that she understands, as I have been very successful each week.

One lady said she has trouble listing her food in the food logbook when she doesn't eat well. I found this to be true. So, to avoid that problem, I stick to the plan that I have written down for the day. I repeat it for about three days before I change something in it, then I follow that new program for another three days.

Just One Bite!

It was getting close to the end of class when the teacher reminded us that previously they had thought it was okay to have a little sweet treat now and then, but they have changed their opinion, as it makes it easier for the person who is trying to lose weight not to take "just one bite." Sugar is like crack cocaine; one little bite will lead to the next little bite, which will lead to the next little bite. Most people can't stop at one little bite. It is the addiction to sugar that the teacher is concerned about. The teachers are very smart, and it is best to learn from these pencils if you are fortunate enough. The teacher said that all it takes is six to eight weeks to get rid of the sugar urge, but I am nervous about that, as I think I could fall in the sugar "crack cocaine" trap very easily with just one little bite, no matter how long it has been since I gave it up.

Shedding My Elephant 2X Skin

A few nights ago I was flipping through the channels. I stopped to watch an animal show from the Buffalo Zoo. Their star elephant took a paintbrush with his trunk, which the trainer had loaded with paint. The elephant took it and brushed it on a two by three foot canvas that was supported by an easel. If an elephant can do THAT, then I can learn better behaviors for myself and thus lose weight. Looking back, it seems like I have been wearing size 2X clothes forever. I am working on shedding that elephant 2X skin to trying on a new graceful giraffe size. Maybe I will transform into another animal size, but if I could choose, I like the grace of the giraffe the best.

If the elephant can paint, then I can transform. There are just three cherry tomatoes sitting on my counter, so I went to the refrigerator and got out my carrots and celery; which is my transformation food.

New Jersey Happiness

Arriving in New Jersey was the beginning of living again without worry. The most devastating thing about not having a job is not knowing when my husband was going to have work again. Often I thought, "If I would just know that in six months we would have a job, then I could let it rest in my mind." The unemployed person doesn't know when tomorrow's job will come. This uncertainty goes on forever until your husband gets that next job.

I turned to comfort food, which is high in carbohydrates. Actually, at the time I didn't even think of it like that. All I thought of was bread and butter, potatoes and pastries, and everything else that could give me comfort. Oh, we ate lots of chickens, but I also ate a lot of the other goodies. The problem I have is that I still see those carbohydrates as delicious. I had one tablespoon of some microwave lasagna last night and I told my husband that it tasted "Out of this world." His response was, "It wasn't really that good." Will I ever shake the delicious carb monkey off my back? I don't know, but I am trying to do my best each day to turn the corner and avoid that monkey.

It was about 10:00 p.m. when the plane landed and midnight when we walked into our hotel room in New Jersey. Next, I had a big surprise. After I took off my shoes and socks, I walked to the bathroom, only to feel water squishing up between my toes. The next day the manager gave us a new room. That night the same thing happened again, and management, who felt bad about our mis-treatment, moved us to the penthouse for the same price as the basic room.

Paradise Is a Warm Swimming Pool and Falling Snow

I didn't spend much time watching the O.J. Simpson civil trial on television, as I used the motel shuttle bus to go over to the Marriott Hotel to swim in their beautiful, window-enclosed pool. I watched the snow falling from the warm water as I did the backstroke. Around me there were patio chairs and large tropical potted plants. It was paradise.

I had what one might call a "food hoarding experience," but at the time it was more of a survival experience. Breakfast was included in the price of the room, but being that I didn't want to eat a large lunch every day in their restaurant, and I was trying to be careful with money, I would take an extra yogurt, wrapped cheese and an apple back to my room after I had eaten breakfast. I did the napkin trick where some of the items disappeared in my purse, but this time it was not due to an addiction. I actually ate that food at noon for lunch after I returned to my motel from swimming.

When David wasn't working we went sightseeing. I feel fortunate that I got to see the Statue of Liberty in New York, Valley Forge in Pennsylvania and the majestic Philadelphia Museum of Art. We went to Princeton University, then rode out to Long Island, where we stopped, at my insistence, to buy a large box of day-old Valentine chocolates. I always looked forward to buying day-old Valentine chocolates, day-old Easter candy and day-old Halloween candy. Now, the day after a holiday, I just walk by those aisles, but I haven't forgotten. Just thinking about chocolate drives me a little crazy.

Learning from Science

"To raise new questions, new possibilities,
to regard old questions from a new angle,
requires creative imagination and marks
real advances in science."
–Albert Einstein

What I like about science is that it educates us. This is not an area where I excel, but it is an area where I can learn. I have tried to collect a few articles about obesity to show the severity of the problem. Twenty to 30 years ago, the severity of the problem was not so pronounced, or was it? Has the media just become more vocal?

From a July 2004 Reader's Digest I found an article titled, "Beating the Urge to Eat," by Peter Jaret, page 118. It starts by saying two dangerously obese children came into a university hospital. They were then given a hormone that controls appetite. [I couldn't believe my eyes when I read something that my teacher had told us. This is another "home run" for my "sharp" teachers.] It said in 1994 a man named Friedman discovered a hormone called leptin. This hormone regulates fat and hunger in our bodies. Many of us get tired in the afternoon, about 3:30, not knowing exactly why. The article says our leptin levels fall and our brain tells us to get something to eat.

When we gain weight our triglyceride level rises. This may prevent leptin from reaching our brain.

Years ago, it was regarded as a willpower problem, but science has discovered that it is much more, and it is a medical problem. Here's to science to come to our rescue and not give us a bad image as just weak individuals.

On June 23, 2010 the University of Buffalo reported, "Baby Tooth Decay Linked to Obesity." Toddlers drink a "sippy" sugar drink. The article said this drink leads to obesity and tooth decay. Not many studies were done connecting these two issues before this study came out. This is the kind of information that mothers can use to give their babies a better life.

There is another article I read, September 12, 2010, entitled "Human Gene Modification Is the Latest Medical Breakthrough on Obesity." Albert Einstein College of Medicine published this study. There is a molecule that affects our hypothalamus, which increases our appetites. Scientists from Imperial College have also done research on this.

On January 5, 2011 there was an article that read, "Childhood Obesity: New Method, New Results." It talks about how children don't go out and play anymore like we did when I was a child, and thus 20 percent of all youngsters in the United States are obese. The article tells about changing the behavior of not only the children, but of the family.

The most recent article I found outlined an area in the southeast of the United States that had the most cases of diabetes. Some of this is economic, and some of it is cultural. I learned how to really increase the calories, and improve the taste of tater tots by frying them when I was in Georgia. Fried food is very popular in the South.

Some have suggested that our government can help by using tax dollars to put in sidewalks where there are none, giving tax credits to people who use gyms to exercise, and to put taxes on high calorie beverages.

People need to help themselves first, and make the effort to lose weight. There is a lot of research being done that can help. Using science is a way toward a better life.

Adventures in China

I got up to take a dill pickle break between writing about science and China. I ate one and it was satisfying. One ounce, which is almost one spear, is only five calories. The sodium is high, but it is only five calories. My world needs to be made of foods that are five calories or less. I decided to use this horizon-

tal pickle bridge to cross over to tell you about my five months in Beijing, China.

We left in the winter six months after we returned from New Jersey. I had packed plenty of my 2X sweaters because I knew it was going to be cold. I also had a few summer clothes, but not nearly enough, as I didn't know how long we would be staying.

We arrived in the early evening. China was a "foreign" world. Passing through customs there was a big long rectangular sign with bold red letters in Chinese. I had no idea what it said, but could tell from the size of the letters, and the boldness of them, that it must be important. A man from the Shangri-La Hotel met us and drove us to the hotel. He wanted to know where we were from. When I said, "Near San Francisco," he said, "Oh yes, near Napa."

This hotel was so posh that each day they changed out the carpets in the elevators to match the day of the week. The breakfast was grand. They had a giant buffet at a giant price of $25 a person. I paid it a few times for myself. David's meals were paid for. Every other day I didn't eat breakfast there to save money. The hotel treated us royally, but it only lasted for a week before the company put us in less luxurious, and less expensive, accommodations.

Later, we moved to the Yanshan Apartments. There was the Modern Plaza nearby, where we could get Western food at expensive prices, but cheaper than $25 for one breakfast. Because of uncertainty of what lay ahead of me, even after reading my tourist books, I brought bags of dried Asian noodles and packages of nutrition bars. I had to have some food for us to eat, at least for the beginning until I could find my way around. I walked one block to the Modern Plaza and for one solid month the construction workers on my route did nothing but stare at me. I had read about this, but knowing it and feeling it are two different things. It was hard on me because I wasn't used to it.

I have a good friend now who helps me with the Chinese language. It is too bad she wasn't with me on the trip. I was paying 60 RMB for a watermelon [Xi (1) Gua (1)] at the Modern Plaza Grocery. At the front desk the lady asked me what they were charging me for one as she saw me bringing them home.

I told her and she was shocked. She told me to bring her a 10 RMB note tomorrow and she would get me one. She walked across the street where there was a small produce stand and bought me a watermelon, while also handing me four RMB in change. She was really nice to me, and helped me in my watermelon purchases all during the time I was there.

I always said hello to everyone, [Ni (2) Ha (3) O], "Knee How" is the phonetic American pronunciation. Once they answered back, I just smiled, not knowing what they said, and even if I did, I had no idea how to answer them.

I had a little Berlitz dictionary with English words listed first, followed by the written Chinese words. There was nothing in this book that said, "The bathroom floor is flooding." After getting out of the tub and standing in two inches of water, I threw on some clothes and raced down the hall to find a maid. I pulled out my book pointing to "the toilet is broken." She could see the distress on my face, and I am sure she noticed as I grabbed her arm motioning for her to come to our apartment. Once she saw the problem, she called on the white service phone near the front door, and within two minutes help arrived. I am not sure of everyone's job, but I know one lady worked at the front desk and two men were plumbers. One man I had seen before, working as their maintenance man. There were a total of nine people in my apartment. Within 45 minutes the problem was fixed. I must say that I have never seen such efficiency and such effort put forth to solve a plumbing problem. If I was in America, it would have taken longer than 45 minutes to get a plumber to my house. The Chinese are very diligent workers. I used to watch them come out each morning and several of them would have their brooms in hand, sweeping the sidewalks and alleys clean.

I went to Tiananmen Square, and also walked a part of the Great Wall. I saw the Summer Palace and the Temple of Heaven. But there is so much more to China than just seeing the tourist attractions.

David and I went out to a nice restaurant once, and standing on a plate on our table was a warrior carved out of a large carrot. We took him home and in order to save him, I put him in the freezer. He stayed in his frozen state for months. When I was ready to take him home to the United States I had a big surprise. After a couple of hours of being out of the freezer he turned into a spongy mess. His sharp carved lines just melted away, so that his "warrior" stature disappeared.

At the Tree House restaurant, we ordered chicken and fish for our group. When this was served, the heads were on the dead animals, including the eyes were looking at us. This was unsettling to me. I had a vegetable dish pronounced "meow," like in a cat's meow, that I really enjoyed.

I had the use of a driver during lhe middle of the day. During the morning and afternoon the driver was for the men to go to work, and to return home from work.

Once I witnessed a man on a bicycle hit our driver's car. The man didn't get hurt. He just ran off in the crowd to disappear somewhere on the other side of the four lane street. Twenty people gathered around our car to talk about the accident. As a passenger I could barely see any daylight because of so many bodies surrounding the car. After a while, our driver told them all to leave, and then he took the man's bicycle and put it in his trunk. The insurance payout for the fender bender was one used bike.

I took many photos of the bikes that I saw in Beijing. China is a land of bikes. I will describe the bikes that I saw by what they carried. There is the "cold soda" bike, the "flattened cardboard" bike, the "fish" bike, the "dung" bike and the "coal" bike. I also saw a "large water bottle" bike, a "wagon" bike, a "pedicab" bike and, of course, just a regular bike.

At the Summer Palace, I read a description of the exhibits in English. Some of them referred to the West, as the "Western Devils." It was written in English so that we would read it.

My experience with the Chinese people is that they either really liked you, or distrusted and disliked you. A man who was head of his choral group at Beihai Park invited me to sing with his group. Three teachers I met at the Chinese Cultural Park were excited to talk to me. I was having trouble crossing a busy four-lane street because the taxi driver let me off on the wrong side of the street. An old man who was selling trinkets saw my problem and put himself in front of me to help me cross the street. One experience that was not as pleasant was when a shy nine year old boy happened to get trapped with us in the apartment elevator. He faced the back corner of the elevator to avoid looking at us. I don't know what terrible things his parents had told him about Westerners, but his reaction was one of sheer panic when he saw us.

I saw many large and beautiful Buddhas. The Reclining Buddha in the Temple of the Reclining Buddha is five meters long and weighs 54 tons. It was made in 1321. Unfortunately, it was plundered during the Cultural Revolution, but was later restored. One special feeling happened to me on this trip. There was a long avenue that was lined with ancient cypress trees that led to the green and yellow tiled entrance. At the entrance to the park I saw a man on a three-wheeled motorcycle that had a passenger seat in the back. He offered to give me a ride to the Temple for a fee, which I paid, even though I could have walked. It seemed like no one was there, so I wasn't taking the seat of an elderly person who might have needed it. As I slowly moved along seated in his powered vehicle I could feel the spring breeze in my hair and see the beautiful trees on each side of this straight as a ruler road. I must confess; I felt like a queen. How grand it was to be charioted down this avenue. Feeling like a queen once in your life, even if it is in a foreign country, sure feels good. After I left the Temple he was waiting for me to take the return trip. The whole experience, my chariot ride, and seeing this majestic Buddha, the first one I had ever seen in a reclining position, was very enriching.

Hamburgers, Watermelon, and Four Bananas Please

Sometimes for lunch I walked across the street to the "A&W All American Food" fast food restaurant, walking past a little stove that had Chinese dumplings, and what looked like lettuce on the table next to the white dumplings. Often the cook wasn't there, but her bike was. The staff at A&W got to know me well. I just ordered by number, as each item was numbered, which was very well thought out because of the foreigners that would come to order food. Hamburgers and watermelon, what a diet.

One time I went out with the boss's wife, a tiny lady, and we saw a man selling bananas. Because of the way that the Chinese fertilize their crops, I felt it best only to eat food where I could peel away the skin. The two of us had our calculators with us, for the merchant to press in the price of what we wanted to buy from him. I held up four fingers indicating that I wanted four bananas. He pressed in a price for us to see and we agreed. I handed over the set price and he handed me three bananas. Then my friend said it again, of course in English, with hand gestures holding up four fingers. She repeated herself again, only speaking a little louder. Then she repeated it again in a still louder voice. At this point, all of the people who were standing around us turned and looked at the "Banana Man," and then he reluctantly handed us the fourth banana that I had paid for. I guess he thought we were dumb tourists, but my friend wouldn't let it go. I arrived home with four bananas in my bag.

The Giant Happy Panda

Later, we moved to the Hui Yuan Apartments. They were originally built as a Chinese Olympic Village. There was a giant smiling panda that I could see looking down from my ninth story window. Once, after I had been there for a while and felt more comfortable with my surroundings, I went down to where the giant panda stood and asked some people if I could take pictures of them. One young man said yes in Chinese, but it was his smile that told me his answer. He then introduced me to his mother, but when I asked to take her picture, she shook her head "No." That was fine with me. I real-

ized that everyone has his own feelings about this. There were many Chinese tourists standing around the panda. Their brief stop at the panda was over and they all returned to their bus. As I stood there watching them, happy that the young man had let me take his photo, something unexpected happened. As I was looking at the side of the bus, every window was full of waving hands, waving goodbye to me.

My Weight Survey

To answer some questions for myself and not depend on a professional survey, I decided to design my own survey. I've never done research like this before. The most unique thing was that some of the participants, including myself, were all in the nude laughing under the showers in the gym while taking the survey. It was fun for all of us. Here are the questions in my survey.

Weight Survey

1) How often do you get on a scale to check your weight?
   a) every hour
   b) every morning and/or every night
   c) once a week
   d) just whenever you feel like it

2) Do you
   a) eat whenever you want to?
   b) watch your food intake careful-ly?

3) Is food
   a) fuel to you?
   b) pleasure to you?

4) When you feel the need to lose weight as in your clothes are getting tight, do you first
   a) reduce your food intake?
   b) increase your physical exercise?
   c) change the types of food you eat?

5) Do you go out to eat
   a) once a day?
   b) once a week?
   c) once a month?
   d) only on birthdays/holidays?
   e) never?

6) If a person is a compulsive drinker, eater, or gambler, can he/she learn not to be compulsive?
   a) yes
   b) no

7) If there were one thing you could change about your physical appearance, what would it be? (This is an essay question for you to answer in your own words on the back of the page.) Thank you very much for taking this survey.

Here are the results for the 21 women who took the survey:

1. How often do you get on the scale to check your weight?
   - 0 a. every hour
   - 4 b. once or twice a day
   - 3 c. once a week
   - 8 d. whenever you feel like it
   - 3 two times per week
   - 1 two times per year
   - 2 no response

2. Do you
   - 11 a. eat whenever you want to
   - 7 b. watch your food intake carefully
   - 3 both a and b

3. Is food
   - 5 a. fuel
   - 11 b. pleasure to you
   - 5 both a and b

4. When you feel you need to lose weight as in your clothes are getting too tight, do you first

3 a. reduce your food intake
2 b. increase your physical exercise
9 c. change the types of food you eat
2 all of the above
1 none of the above
2 buy bigger clothes
2 does not apply

5. Do you go out to eat

2 a. once a day
10 b. once a week
4 c. once a month
1 d. only on birthdays/holidays
0 e. never
1 three to four times a week
2 one to two times a week
1 one to two times a month

6. If a person is a compulsive drinker, eater, or gambler, can he/she learn not to be compulsive?
   16 a. yes
   3 b. no
   1 don't know
   1 no response

7. If there were one thing you could change about your physical appearance, what would it be?
   8 be fit and slim
   2 lose weight
   1 be taller
   1 have plastic surgery
   1 have larger breasts
   1 have smaller breasts
   1 change hair style
   1 be younger
   5 no response

Fifty percent of the women said they just eat whenever they want, and 50 percent of the women regard food as pleasure. My biggest surprise was the prevailing attitude that a person can learn not to be compulsive. I don't agree with this. I think the compulsive behavior is just redirected in another way.

For myself, I did a before and after quiz. It makes me think of the before and after photos that a person sees in a home beautiful magazine. First you see the barren bedroom before, and then you see the bedroom with a new coat of paint. In the second photo you see new furniture adorned with colorful pillows.

Here is my "Before Survey," before I even tried to lose weight.

1 – I weighed myself whenever I felt like it.

2 – I ate whenever I wanted to.

3 – Food was pleasure for me.

4 – I would buy larger clothes when the current ones I was wearing got too tight.

5 – I went out to eat every day, eating whatever I wanted.

6 – I thought a person could learn not to be compulsive.

7 – The one thing I wanted was to become thinner.

Now you see the "After Survey," taken after working hard and having lost 20 pounds.

1 – I weigh myself every Tuesday morning.

2 – I watch my food intake carefully.

3 – Food is fuel to me now; this makes me a little sad.

4 – I reduce my food intake when I notice that my clothes are getting a little tight.

5 – I still go out to eat once a day, but I check the menu to get a low calorie option.

6 – I believe a person cannot change from being compulsive.

7 – I know I can lose weight now, so I wish to be as beautiful as I can be.

I surprised myself on my answer to number seven. I was sure I would say I wanted to be thinner. When you have a grasp on something, you no longer have the obsessive desire to get it. I know I will have to work on this the rest of my life, but I have finally given myself the power to do it.

Help Wanted: Grocery Store Courage

I know I have to work on my attitude about food and get a more positive frame of mind, which I learned from taking my weight survey. Going to the grocery store makes me feel sad. It is like going to an electronics store, where there are just a few things that I could buy. All I feel at the grocery store is that I am loading my cart with gasoline. Often I look straight down the row with my eyes parallel to the tile strip on the floor. I make sure to keep my eyes focused straight ahead of me so as not to bump into anyone. Toward the right and left I can see in my peripheral vision pasta, ice cream, cakes, nuts and potato salad. If there is something I can't find I prefer to let it go, rather than scan each row looking for it. That just increases my pain. I am learning in my mind that I don't want to eat many of those foods, but in my heart, I often still feel the way I did before. It is a tug of war between the two.

The dilemma is to stay fat and get fatter because that is what happens to me when I eat (I think food compounds itself like interest over the years), or to live in a mechanical world where going to the grocery store is equivalent to going to the gas station. It is something I will have to live with, but I doubt many overweight people do this, only those that are trying to lose weight. There are more options for me that could be considered: I could send my husband to the store, or I could order groceries online. In either case, I wouldn't have to walk down the grocery store aisles.

"Just Half a Cup of Pasta!"
–Alice

Seven people were in class today. We discussed "Exercise," and "Burning Calories." By just sitting we are burning one calorie a minute, but when we are doing vigorous exercise we are burning much more.

Also discussed was how the brain only uses carbohydrates to work. I did the Atkins diet in San Diego, and I did lose weight, but I found it impossible to stay on this diet due to my extreme headaches.

The teacher handed out a quiz on different aspects of things we have learned in the class. I let the other six answer the questions, as they seemed more eager to do so. There were questions about cardio and weight lifting, and nothing about walking and swimming, so I kept quiet.

The food questions are more applicable to me. One question went all the way back to the second or third class: How much is a USDA serving of pasta? The answer is half a cup of cooked pasta. This answer ruffled the feathers of some of the students. Alice asked, "How can anybody eat just half a cup of pasta?" She's right. I can't, so I just won't eat pasta. The problem is resolved for me. This following sentence is all in caps, as it is so important. ONCE YOU GET OFF YOUR STRUCTURED PLAN, YOU WILL PUT THE WEIGHT BACK ON.

We were told that a meal should hold us for four hours and a snack for two. The women in the class were talking about how hard it is to tell the waiter to take the rolls/bread away from the table. Then the teacher said, "Yes, but it is even harder to have the bread sitting on the table with you looking at it." Oh, this is so true.

Also discussed was the fact that the longer you survive without chocolate the longer you don't want it anymore. Come to think of it, chocolate is sort of fading away in my brain. I know I used to really like it, and if I was to taste it again, I bet I would like it, but I will just keep my memory of chocolate melting away in my brain.

A Mile for a Muffin

Our second teacher talked about an article in Time Magazine, August 17, 2009, by John Cloud entitled, "Why Exercise Won't Make You Thin." It said that exercise often stimulates hunger, and that is when the person goes out and rewards herself with a muffin. So she burned 300 calories, but she is going to blow it by eating the muffin. Most likely the muffin is going to be more than 300 calories, so in the weight game, she has lost. I am not sure if men have this mentality, but I know women do.

The article says exercise does have other beneficial effects, which are mental health and prevention of heart disease, but the author stresses that he doubts exercise is effective in weight loss. I admire the teacher's courage for sharing this article with us. One lady in the class has really been exercising. They see her in the gym almost every day. She hasn't lost any weight.

Often people over estimate just how much the exercise is worth. For example, is that one-hour worth a large muffin? After we mowed the lawn, as I put my cup of water in the microwave to heat for some tea, I joked with my husband and said, "This is my muffin treat." We both laughed.

The teacher discussed how overweight people often overeat, even after they are full, but that normal weight people only overeat occasionally. A good workout does help you mentally, and thus can help mildly depressed people.

The teacher said that people who keep the weight off have some type of exercise for 60 minutes a day. Many are walkers. My goal is to do what I can that will not increase my hunger, and do an exercise that will not cause a sports injury. Walking works for me. Doing enough exercise will take a lot of adjustment for me. I know I am not there yet, but I am walking in the right direction.

Land of 17,508 Islands

Indonesia is a Pacific Ocean nation in Southeast Asia that consists of over 17,000 islands. It is the largest Muslim country in the world. I lived on Java and Batam over a period of more than two years. I studied about this country before we left, but book knowledge is not the same as the knowledge you acquire by living in a country.

We were briefly in Jakarta, mostly to travel to and from the airport. Once there was some business to be taken care of, and another time we went shopping at an expensive store. For this trip, our driver dropped us off right at the front door of the department store, and we agreed on three in the afternoon for him to pick us up at the same place where he had dropped us off. He told us this was for our safety, because it was not good to be waiting around in front of the department store.

Indonesia was a colony of the Netherlands, but in 1949 the Dutch finally recognized Indonesia's independence. Mentos, which is a mint candy that originated in the Netherlands, still sits on merchants' shelves. I loved eating this candy that kept me going during the long afternoons between lunch and dinner. Here is how it went. I ate one after another after another, and stopped about 30 minutes before dinner so as to have a good appetite.

We first lived on the island of Java in a town called Bogor, about 60 kilometers south of Jakarta. This area had a rural atmosphere and thus I was sheltered from seeing Indonesia's poverty. It is a country rich in natural resources, and those profits went into the "elites" hands, thus poverty remains widespread in Indonesia. I later saw with my own eyes, after living there for a while and venturing out, how extensive the poverty was.

The Frog and the Tiger

We stayed at the Novotel Bogor in a lovely ground floor room that had an outdoor Jacuzzi for bathing. High bushes for privacy surrounded our room. Not knowing anyone, not even the staff, I watched the funeral of

King Hussein of Jordan who died on February 7, 1999. Briefly I saw Queen Noor of Jordan. She was renamed after her conversion to Islam. She used to be Elizabeth Najeeb Halaby. She was a strikingly beautiful woman with blonde hair. She wasn't allowed to see her husband at the funeral, and I thought this was so sad.

A baby frog got trapped in the corner of our room, and once at night I thought I heard a tiger on the other side of the glass door separating our sleeping area from the Jacuzzi. It was just a cat, but in my dream, it sounded like a tiger. A colleague of David's once found a poisonous snake in the shower stall of his room.

Island Mountain Fear

It was while staying here that I heard the frightening stories from the expat wives about things that happened in Jakarta. One lady told me she never takes her passport with her, as she was robbed while in a taxi, and all of the contents in her purse were lost.

I was also told to watch out for the taxi driver's trick, where he stops on the corner to pick up one other passenger, who then robs you and runs from the cab. That evening the driver meets with his friend, the robber, and they split the loot. Fear engulfed me. How was I ever going to leave the hotel?

The hotel celebrated "Idul Fitri" while we were there. This occurs after the month-long period of Ramadan, during which Muslims fast from dawn until sunset. Ramadan is when they purify themselves, and ask forgiveness for past sins. At the end of this month-long fast is a celebration called "Idul Fitri," the festival of breaking the fast.

Idul Fitri is a special celebration. I remember working with the staff making little paper and ribbon packets. These were symbolic for the packets that would contain cooked rice. Everyone was so happy that Idul Fitri was coming in a few days.

Deer Roaming At the Presidential Palace

Once, during our month long stay here, I went sightseeing with a foreign businesswoman who made frequent trips to Jakarta. We went to see the "Istana Bogor" which is their large Presidential Palace. It was built in 1744 as a retreat for the Dutch Governors. What was most unusual about this place was that in the fenced grounds there were many, many deer roaming around the lawn. This custom was preserved, even though the Indonesians did not eat deer meat after the Dutch left. Extended families who were picnicking near the royal grounds waved to us. This was clearly a happy place. I always took a couple of rolls of Mentos with me, just to make sure I didn't get hungry.

On another trip, our driver took us along Puncak Pass to see a tea plantation, which was between Jakarta and Bandung. I saw a sign that celebrates the joy of drinking tea. I personally love tea, but drank a lot of ice tea because of the tropical temperatures.

"Tea"

If you are Cold, TEA will warm you
If you are too heated, IT will cool you
If you are depressed, IT will cheer you
If you are excited, IT will calm you.

–W.F. Gladstone, 1865

Saved By Carrots

Reviewing my activities I realized we must have been in this location longer than a month. One fun weekend trip was to Taman Safari Indonesia. We drove around and saw the elephants, the giraffes and the camels.

There was a brief stop where we all did a little walking. I was walking down a gentle slope with a colleague of my husband beside me. My camera was hanging around my neck, so no one could use it to take a photo of me. All of a sudden, a large orangutan walked up from behind us and placed one hand on my left arm. The other hand he placed on Oscar's right arm. The orangutan walked upright like a human, so perfectly that I thought perhaps he was a man in a Disney orangutan suit.

As we walked I noticed, looking down at his arm, how perfect every hair was. It was truly amazing for a costume. Then it hit me. What man has the powerful grip that I was feeling on my arm? I realized then that he was a real orangutan, and I'd still be connected to him today if he hadn't eyed the carrots his trainer had set out for him. One amazing thing about the orangutan is that he didn't put his hand over my watch. That was another thing that fooled me into thinking maybe he was a man in a costume. The truth is that he was just a well-trained orangutan.

I was clearly not in shape when we walked to see the crater at the bottom of the "Tangkuban Parahu" mountain. I never re-

ally made it to the bottom, as my legs felt like rubber. I sat on a rock two-thirds of the way down while my husband and one colleague went all the way down. Several thin, strong, short Indonesian men helped me to get back up to the parking lot.

Every evening we dined at the hotel restaurant and I became friends with the workers. I took a lot of photos of them, and on a return trip two years later, I gave them all photos of themselves. I never did experiment much with food, but always chose a chef salad or a club sandwich because I felt more comfortable with this. David did experiment. You might think that my adventurous spirit would have extended to food, but it didn't.

My Blue Ribbon Exercise-Calisthenics

In the late afternoon in Batam, after the worst heat of the day but before dinner, I would do water exercises in their football field size pool. Somehow, even though I didn't get that much exercise, I was able to maintain my weight in Indonesia. When I think about it, with all the sewing I did, and all the candy I ate while I was sewing, I guess I feel fortunate that I didn't gain any weight.

I wish I had known about my newly adopted Blue Ribbon exercise when I was abroad. In China, at each place we lived, there was no pool and these calisthenics would have come in handy. I'll use them in all my future travels. Thank you, pencil number three, for sharing this information with the class. I am slow at these exercises, but I am starting to MOVE again.

Eleven Quilts in Two Years

Many women do not travel with their husbands on extended stays in foreign countries. Often, the reason is as simple as their having children in school. David and I discussed the possible trip to Batam, Indonesia, but I reminded him that many days while he was working, there were times in Bogor when I got bored simply because there was not enough to do. Reading books and going to their pool didn't fill a whole day. I found out that the hardest thing to do is to have nothing to do.

We decided David should take the job in Batam. Batam is a free trade zone, just 12 miles from Singapore. We figured we could buy a sewing machine for me in Singapore to make quilts. There were stores on Batam, but not having been there, I didn't know what was actually available.

Nagoya is the biggest town in Batam and features many stores. Industries on this island are shipbuilding and electronics manufacturing. There are also several resorts. In

2006 Batam was made into a "Special Economic Zone with Singapore." By doing this, tariffs and special value-added taxes were eliminated for goods shipped between Batam and Singapore. I often wondered what the customs officials thought when they saw an American couple walking through the line with a portable sewing machine. My guess is that not many people did this.

The Western Side of Paradise

At the first hotel where we stayed in Nagoya, Batam, I felt a little uncomfortable, without really knowing why. About a week later I noticed, as I looked over the mezzanine into the lobby below, that men were waiting there as women came in wearing fancy clothes met them, and then the men escorted them out. This wasn't just one man, but several, and it happened on several occasions.

A co-worker of David's who was in Batam only briefly found another place to stay, and as I was having lunch with his wife, I found out the name of this other hotel. Shortly after this, we moved to "Waterfront City."

It was a much nicer place for me to live, where I could feel comfortable. I was a bird in a gilded cage. On some occasions, David would pick me up and we would go into Nagoya to have lunch at the two story McDonalds. Only foreigners ate there. The cost of the meal was so high that it would have been excessive for an Indonesian family to afford.

Sitting next to the window on the second floor, I could see the beggars on the street. Some were crippled. Once I saw a child asleep on the sidewalk only to see a businessman kick the sleeping child's arm out of his path where he was walking. It disturbed me to see how callous some people can be. The child wasn't in school because his parents didn't have enough money to send him.

The Road to Buddhist Beauty

To break up the monotony of living in paradise, I went on a tour offered by the hotel. The only problem was that it was for Chinese speaking people. I didn't care, as I just wanted to get out and see some of the surroundings. The first stop was to a seafood restaurant on a long pier. Eating what everyone else was eating was fine with me, until I heard John Denver on a CD, singing "Almost Heaven, West Virginia." I had trouble keeping tears from my eyes, as I gazed at the scenery beyond the water.

On the trip we saw a temple and some Buddhas at the temple. We also saw a tourist amusement area where they had ice-skating, but it had closed down and we all sat on the benches that were outside this building. The bus driver took a little rest, before one last stop.

Our last stop was the Indonesia Maitreya Missionary, an educational compound for those studying to be Buddhist monks. All of the students there were friendly to me, even though I wasn't Buddhist. To me it was the most peaceful place on the island, and a place that brought me much serenity. Later, I often came by myself with a taxi to visit this haven of tranquility.

In the hotel one man was trying to pursue me, but his motives were not honest, as he was much younger than I. Why would he be interested in an overweight 50 year old woman? Often, when I saw him coming from a distance, I hid my face behind an open newspaper, as he made me feel uncomfortable.

For exercise and recreation I would go to the hotel pool. Once I saw two boisterous British men attempting to court an Indonesian *woman, only to see them the next day with bodies red like radishes. There was a nice pool bar in the middle of the pool and occasionally I would order something to eat, like chicken legs and a soda.*

"Kirsten, Move Your Arm"
–A Singapore Doctor

I did vigorous water exercises, and one morning when I awoke, I couldn't move my left arm. We called David's sister who is a nurse wondering if she had any idea what was wrong with me. Naturally, without seeing me, and on the little information that I gave her, she couldn't make any diagnosis. We quickly left the hotel and were on our way to Singapore to see a doctor. I couldn't move my arm so much as a fraction of an inch without pain. Just to make the trip, because I was in so much pain, I know I took too many Motrin.

Our regular doctor in Singapore made an appointment at the hospital for the next morning, as it was already 3:30 p.m. The next day the specialist gave me a cortisone shot in my shoulder as I lay there. He used a big TV like monitor to spot the exact location where he should give me the injection. After-

wards the doctor said, "Kirsten, move your arm." I said, "No, I can't." He said, "Let me help you," and then without pain I saw out of the corner of my eye that my arm was no longer resting on the table. What had happened to me was called "frozen shoulder."

On other occasions we had several fun trips to Singapore. Each trip cost us $200 to $300, but it was our relaxation treat. We walked along Clarke Quay and saw un art exhibit called, "Monet to Moore" at one of the art museums. We saw Chinatown where I photographed a red cabinet that had butterfly handles, with one wing on each side of the door. It was here that we saw a Hindu temple with concrete cows sitting on the roof. The National Orchid Garden was so beautiful, but on such a hot, humid day some of the beauty was lost to me.

Yellow Rice Brings Good Luck

Returning to the hotel in the evening after riding on the ferry and going through customs at both ends, Singapore and Indonesia, we enjoyed our evening at the "Long Stay Guest Party" in April 1999. We didn't receive any prizes, as we hadn't been there long enough.

The food display was artistic. My thoughts were, "How in the world can anybody eat this?" There was a large honeydew melon with the rind removed and decorated to look like a face. Placed on the melon were two large cherry pupil eyes, and red and yellow pepper strips placed around the eyes. The strips were also used to form a nose and a mouth. There were five palm branches on top of the melon to complete this tribal dancer look. It is hard to explain, but at parties in Indonesia, I saw men dressed in costumes wearing animal masks as they danced. This honeydew melon artwork reminded me of those dancers. At the bottom of its face were lines of cut up watermelon, pineapple, and mango for the guests to eat. There was also a large bowl of yellow rice. I was told if I ate some yellow rice it would bring me good luck. For entertainment, the hotel had women dancers in native costumes. It was a grand party.

Riot in Nagoya

We were living at Waterfront City, away from the town of Nagoya. Once, when we returned to Batam from Singapore, we found that the other Americans had left. The island had become a ghost town. The stores in Nagoya were closed. During our trip to Singapore, two immigrant groups had clashed, fighting over the control of a bus route.

Nine people had died. We heard stories that people were running around with two by fours with nails sticking from them for protection. One Indonesian man we knew stayed up all night placing lumber on the inside of his front door to guard his property. It was after this skirmish that the hotel director told me that he had an evacuation plan for his guests. About 50 feet from our hotel we could board a boat to get to Singapore and out of danger.

A Special American Thanksgiving in Indonesia

There was another grand party that David and I attended. After about six months of being in Indonesia I met another American, Pauline, who became one of my best friends. Her husband managed one of the electronics factories in Batam. She was more adventurous than I was, and rented a house, whereas I lived in a hotel for over two years. She had been in Indonesia for seven years and knew a lot of the language.

The people of the town really had respect for her. She had passed out "gift packages" at Christmas to many of the families who lived near her. She had a driver and a manservant as well as a maid. Every time she went home to America she gave them gifts when she returned. Her heart is made of gold.

The week before Thanksgiving she went to Singapore and bought a large turkey to bring back to Batam. For the holiday she prepared a feast for her expatriate friends that included pumpkin pie, custard pie, mashed potatoes, succotash, sweet potatoes with marshmallows, egg noodles and rice. She also made brownies. Her hospitality magically turned Indonesia into America for that day.

A Friend to the People of Her Village

Before I knew Pauline she had worked on setting up a grade school in her village. She bought all the supplies for her school.

Once, some robbers attempted to break into her house at 3:00 a.m. Her manservant hid under the bed, but the driver ran up the hill to ring the "community bell" that announced danger. All the townspeople that lived around her rushed to her aid. This scared the robbers, who saw the flood of people running toward the house. Nothing was taken; the robbers ran away in fright. The people that she knew in Indonesia loved her. I feel honored to have known her.

The German Diet

Writing about the grand Thanksgiving we had with Pauline made me think of the delicious German food we ate when I was growing up. We were all American at home; we spoke English; we dressed like Americans; and we associated with other Americans. At first Mutti went to an "International Club" that had several Germans in it, but after a few meetings she left. She said they were "too stuck up," and she didn't like that attitude. From the very beginning I integrated with the Americans around me, as did my parents. One part of me did stay German, though. That was my diet.

The two activities I did was going to school and playing. I can remember wrapping up my Honey Baby doll in a blanket and getting a few supplies, such as her bottle and a change of clothes, to take her to preschool with me. But I never remembered what was on the dinner table each night. I can remember our Christmas morning breakfast the best.

I can tell you some of the foods we ate, and especially some of the foods my father ate. I was always picky with food. When our Uncle Quincy came to visit us from Brownsville, Texas, he would take us out to eat at a steak house. My mother would order scrambled eggs for me. He'd often bring us a basketful of large, beautiful red grapefruit. Uncle Quincy would always take me to the store and let me buy a doll. I got a cute little girl Easter bunny once. To be truthful, that is what I remember, not the food.

Back to the food: My father ate asparagus as well as dark pumpernickel bread. We never had a black forest cake, which is a chocolate cake with white icing and some cherries on top. I tasted this dessert for the first time when I went on a trip with Mutti to visit her sister, Aunt Iris, who lived close to the Black Forest. I do remember when my Aunt Iris sent me Christmas packages containing Lebkuchen, a spicy gingerbread flavored cookie, which I have always loved.

We often ate potatoes and sausages. Many times we couldn't get sausages, so we ate hot dogs because that is what we could get at Piggly Wiggly. My father made the best potato salad. It had mustard, egg and mayonnaise in it, in addition to the potatoes. No cookbook was ever used, as it was a taste as you go project. At the end he would figure out if it needed more salt, more mustard, or if it was too dry and needed a little more water.

We didn't eat dumplings, as that took more preparation to make. Mutti worked as well as my father and there just wasn't enough time to do elaborate cooking. For Thanksgiving, my father bought some prepared chicken to take home and eat. He felt my mother worked hard and she should enjoy the day off from work.

Bratwurst has always been a favorite of mine, but really I can't remember it from my childhood. Here is a list of ingredients:

- 6 slices bacon
- 1 small onion, chopped
- 1 clove garlic, minced
- 1 can of sauerkraut (32 oz.), drained and rinsed
- 2 medium potatoes, peeled and sliced
- 1 cup water
- 1/2 cup white grape or apple juice
- 1 Tablespoon brown sugar

- 1 cube chicken bouillon
- 1 bay leaf
- 1 teaspoon caraway seed
- 1 pound bratwurst
- 1 large apple, cored and sliced

Another favorite at our house was rye bread. This was dressed up with mustard containing horseradish, and layered with cheese or sandwich meat.

Many people in Germany eat Kartoffelknödeln (potato dumplings). Here are the ingredients:

- 8 medium potatoes
- 3 egg yolks, beaten
- 3 Tablespoons cornstarch
- 1 cup bread crumbs
- 1/2 teaspoon pepper
- 1-1/2 teaspoon salt
- Flour

One favorite I made after moving away from home, not even realizing that it was German, is Apfelpfannkuchen (apple pancakes). To me, they were always called apple pancakes. Here is a list of ingredients:

- 2/3 cup flour
- 2 teaspoons sugar

- 1/4 teaspoon salt
- 4 eggs, beaten
- 1/2 cup milk
- 2 large apples, peeled, cored and cut into thin slices
- 1-1/2 sticks of butter (3/4 cup)
- 2 tablespoons sugar
- 1/4 teaspoon cinnamon
- Confectioners' sugar

With the evening meal Mutti always served frozen peas and carrots, or canned sauerkraut, whatever she could get at the store.

On Christmas morning we ate brown and serve rolls with jam. There was also a plate on the table that had meat and cheese on it. This was for our second helping.

My food was rich and very full of calories, but that is my heritage. I still love that food, but because I want more than just a few bites, I'll have to stay away from it. I will tell you that it's very hard to adjust in your 60s to eating different foods, but I know that I must, and I like how I feel weighing 20 pounds less.

The French Diet

Next I have a diet from a French lady. My guess is that she weighs around 120 pounds. She is very thin. I asked her to write down what she eats during the day.

Breakfast

- 1 big glass of water (room temperature or warm)
- Green tea (all morning long, 1-2 quarts)
- Go Lean 13g protein cereals (1 cup)
- Ground flaxseed (3 tsp)
- Almond Granola (3 tsp)

And depending on my appetite

- 1 or 2 slices of whole wheat bread with preserves or light cheese

Lunch

- Grilled meat or fish (no fat)
- 1 or 2 eggs
- Steamed vegetables, or sautéed vegetables in olive oil
- A piece of cheese (if very hungry)
- A cup of plain non-fat yogurt and granola (if hungry)

- Or a few cookies
- One or two squares of 72 percent dark chocolate

Snack

- One piece of fresh fruit (apple, banana, or orange)

Dinner

- A large plate of pasta and herbs, or rice, or quinoa, or potatoes (no meat)
- A cup of applesauce
- A piece of bread or a cookie

She told me she doesn't drink water during meals, but only between meals and never ice water. She said she drinks a glass of wine when she has guests over. She also said she never goes to bed hungry. She exercises seven days a week for 45 minutes each session. Looking at her you would never believe that she has arthritis, and has had a hip replacement. She is in better shape and health than I am. I'm amazed at all she eats. I am wondering if I should change over to a French diet. Where I would fall short is that I don't exercise like she does. I do think that as more and more of my fat melts away I will be able to exercise more. Let's just hope that happens.

The Chinese Diet

Two Chinese ladies, both thin and beautiful, talked to me about their diets. I asked them each what they ate.

Breakfast

- 1 Cup of Milk
- 1 Large Slice of Bread (from a Chinese bakery)
- 1/2 apple

Lunch

- 1 medium bowl of rice – or a salad

Dinner

- 1 small bowl of rice
- 1 large plate of Chinese cooked vegetables

She told me she doesn't eat much meat, and that she swims laps five times a week. She came to America when she was 22 years old. Her first year here she gained 30 pounds because of all the ice cream, chocolate and burgers that she ate. She admitted that American food is delicious, but she did lose those 30 pounds and went back to her Asian diet. She told me that she eats up to the point where she feels about 70 percent full.

Another Chinese friend told me that she usually doesn't go to bed hungry. Here is what she eats.

Breakfast

- Garlic bread – a 4 inch piece

Lunch

- Two Cups of rice
- One Cup of cooked vegetables
- Scrambled eggs with tomatoes

Dinner

- 10 boiled dumplings

Twice a week she goes to the gym. She has a job that takes a lot of her time; otherwise I think she would love to go more frequently to exercise. Her brother and mother are larger than she is. She has her father's thin build. When she is stressed she scarcely eats any food. [I should be doing this.] She told me she is happy that she is not fat. She thinks weight is related to the genetics in your family. I was amazed when she told me that there are some large Chinese ladies who are in the Line Dancing Class.

Asian diets are usually rich in rice, fish and vegetables. They limit dairy and meat (although pork is very popular). Very little sweets are ever eaten. Once in Beijing I went to a bakery and purchased an item that was wrapped in dough. I expected a sweet cinnamon taste, only to be surprised that inside was some sort of paste that tasted strange.

A lot of cooked vegetables are eaten in China. One lady I know told me that when she goes on this type of Eastern diet, she doesn't count her calories and she has noticed that she doesn't gain any weight. Some people think that the Western diet, which has too much sugar, wheat and meat, is the cause of diabetes, cardiovascular disease and obesity. I am eating more vegetables now, learning from my Chinese friends.

The Indian Diet

India is a big country of several languages, religions, music and dance. Even today, as has been the tradition, several generations often live in the same household, while some Indian families have adopted a nuclear family structure.

Many Indian people have a vegetarian diet. The lady who shared her diet with me told me she was a vegetarian. She eats some Western foods, as she has lived in America for many years. The menu she wrote for me is a varied sample. Not all the items listed under "Dinner," are served at each meal, but generally, she told me that they put one lentil curry on the table with one curried vegetable dish, along with rice, chapattis and plain yogurt. Here is a typical day of an Indian/American diet.

Breakfast

- Two slices of whole wheat toast with jelly (jam)
- A bowl of steel-cut oatmeal with vanilla soy milk
- A banana with yogurt

Lunch

- A spinach salad
- A sandwich (vegetarian burger)

Dinner

- Half a cup of steamed white rice
- Two whole wheat chapattis (similar to whole wheat tortilla)
- Half a cup of cooked lentils (brown, black, green, yellow)
- Half a cup cooked vegetables

An Indian friend in our neighborhood gave me this traditional diet from Northern, Central and Western India:

Breakfast

- Parantha (plain or stuffed with herbs etc.) and yogurt
- Milk or tea
- Pickles
- Lassi (yogurt based drink)

Lunch and Dinner

- Roti and rice
- Fresh vegetables
- Lentils
- Kidney beans, chickpeas
- Yogurt, salad
- Indian sweets

Late Afternoon or Evening Snack

- Warm tea
- Samosas (a stuffed pastry)

I am so fortunate to have these good friends. They talk to me like I am not fat. Their loving eyes look beyond my size as they tell me about their diets and their stories. The world is a better place when more people do this.

We just returned from the grocery store. I am getting brave. Since my new meal plan is for the rest of my life, I wore a new face in the grocery store. I felt proud as we walked through the produce section and thought to myself, "These foods are good for me, they are going to make me healthier." I have decided that I am going to be positive, and not feel sorry for myself. I am going to really work hard in my venture to lose weight.

Tip # 13
"As a man thinketh in his heart, so is he."
–Book of Proverbs, Chapter 23, Verse 7, The Bible

As I change my attitude to be more positive, then the results that follow will be more positive. I am walking out of my old life into my new one, pound by pound.

Alligators to Zebras – What Do They Eat?

Just for the fun of it, I did a little research on animals and their food consumption. Hummingbirds eat more than their weight each day. They eat 14 times an hour, otherwise they could starve.

Crocodiles seldom need to eat, as they are cold blooded and have a low metabolism. Tigers can eat as much as 40 pounds of meat at a time. After this feast they do not eat again for several days.

I guess my point is that animals can regulate themselves better, so what is wrong with man? How did we get so far off the track? I've switched tracks now, and may my life be better for it.

Super Food Beads You Eat

In class we were introduced to baby kiwi, and a food that I didn't know about called quinoa. The food dictionary, Epicurus, says it is new to the American diet. It was a staple of the ancient Incas. As I was eating the sample given to me I noticed it consisted of tiny, bead-like pebbles. Quinoa has a reputation for being a super food, as it contains complete protein. The teacher calls it power food. Of all the food that we were given to sample, this one was my favorite, and I could have easily asked for a second helping.

The freeze-dried fruit didn't appeal to me. It tasted like an apple flavored potato chip. Irving really liked it, so I gave him mine. The teacher said that lentils are "powerhouses," but they are high in calories.

Students in the class are trying to get more vegetables in their diet. I do this too. I'm lazy as I don't like to cook them. I buy the already washed ones, and eat them straight from the bag. I really don't think that I have the excitement about food that I once had. Some students are choosing to eat smaller portions and eliminate the junk food. One lady brought up that when she is out of her element, like on vacation or at a restaurant, food choices seem to get out of control. This is something that happens to me. I have been staying away from these situations until I can learn to handle them better.

The class ended promptly at the end of the hour, and all the ladies disappeared into the night, like ashes in a fireplace when a new log is thrown on top. I wonder if at the end of all the weight classes, a weight loss friend will be around for me.

I have learned that the moment I see my weight creeping back on, I have to start recording exactly what I eat. This helps pull me in line, so that the advancing weight won't take control.

Like the other women in the class, I feel there is the struggle between what to feed your family, and what to feed yourself. I could never handle this. My children have left home now, and my husband supports me in my weight loss efforts. Even though I have been shedding the pounds, actually grating them off is a better word, my heart is still large and full of compassion to help any overweight person who wants my help. Love is more powerful than a calorie. Don't be fooled by the thinner body, my heart is just the same as before.

One woman brought up the fact that she just likes to eat. I understand. Family celebrations seem to focus on food, which is another reason that it is so difficult for many people to lose weight. After the party is over, they can't seem to go back to watching their calories again.

Like so many other people, I love to eat. I have dieted many times and gained the weight back because I love to eat. The taste of wonderfully cooked food excites me. Eating is one of the joys that accompany family rituals, like holidays, birthdays, anniversaries and weddings. Often I have met friends and we visited together during a delicious lunch. I remember going to a bakery and having a sandwich to go with a sweet treat. These times are special occasions where we have fun being with each other and eating.

Some of my best memories center on food. At the first Christmas celebration with my son and his new wife, we sang "Silent Night" in English and then in Portuguese. My daughter-in-law made her famous Brazilian chicken/crust/cheese mouthwatering entrée while I brought my favorite Lebkuchen ginger/chocolate coated cookies for dessert. We also had my father's potato salad, my daughter's sweet potatoes and chocolate pecan pie, and my son's signature hearts of palm garden salad, as well as some celery and cherry tomatoes for Christmas color. The table effervesced with goodness and the family that stood around it was so happy to be there. These are the best times to remember.

Bangers and Mash in Indonesia

Welcome back to Batam, Indonesia. Sometimes, but only with my husband or a group of people, I went into Nagoya. A few times we went to Lucy's Oarhouse, a pub that features fish and chips, bangers and mash, and hamburgers. They sell a T-shirt that says, "Lucy's Rock Hard Café, Nagoya, Batam."

There was a grand party on Indonesia's Independence Day, August 17. Again, we had magnificent displays of food before us. Artistic palm trees were made of carrots topped with hollowed out green peppers. Girls dressed in native costumes. Most of the staff of the hotel was there.

I came, and in my own simple way, paid respect to their country. In my hair I wore two large spools of thread, one was red and the other was white. Both were tied on the top of my head with a shoelace. The hotel employees were happy and placed me between them as David took a photo of us.

Christmas Eve Bombings

On Christmas Eve, while the hotel was playing a lot of loud music, a series of explosions took place in different cities in Indonesia. It was written up in Wikipedia that Al Qaeda and Jemaah Islamiyah were responsible for bombing Christian churches. Three bombs went off in a church in Batam, injuring 22 people. My friend, Pauline narrowly escaped the bombing, having left the church 15 minutes before the explosion. All this happened while we were sitting around the pool listening to music, eating, drinking and celebrating Christmas Eve.

For New Years 2000, there was another party with music, food and fireworks outdoors under the moonlight. At the end of the party, David and I danced on the beach to welcome in the new century.

Y2K Is Approaching

The month of December had a couple of things that made it different. There was the panic over the Year 2000 problem (also known as the Y2K problem) along with the Christmas Eve bombings that I mentioned before. This Y2K "Millennium Bug" meant that there were going to be gigantic problems with computer programs. This is the problem as I understand it: The issue is the "rollover" from 1999 (X99 to X00). Some data could be processed incorrectly, and this could have disastrous effects. There is some dispute over how many computer failures occurred, but from what I understand the transition went rather smoothly.

The Nasi Goreng Winner

The hotel had another party early in the year. They had a "Nasi Goreng" contest. This is one of the best-known rice dishes of Indonesia. I, along with a few other expatriates, played in the game. The challenge was to make the best Nasi Goreng dish. Please review this recipe before proceeding. I am listing the ingredients:

Nasi Goreng - Indonesian Fried Rice

- 4 cups cold cooked rice

- 2 Tablespoons oil
- 1 egg, lightly beaten
- 5 shallots, peeled and sliced
- 2 cloves garlic, peeled and sliced
- 3 red chilies sliced
- 1 teaspoon dried shrimp paste
- ½ teaspoon salt
- 1 Tablespoon sweet soy sauce
- Sliced cucumbers (to garnish)
- 8 oz. sliced chicken, sliced pork, or medium shrimp
- 1 cup shredded cabbage (optional)

The food preparation table was set with rice, vegetables and spices. A chef judged all the entries as to their authenticity. I took my plate, plopped a bunch of rice on it, took a few cucumbers to make it pretty and then plopped a fried egg on top. Everywhere we went in Indonesia when David ordered Nasi Goreng it was served with a fried egg on top. That part I did correctly.

What happened next is unbelievable. After the chef had finished judging, the awards were given out. I was honored when he came over and gave me first prize. The hotel staff really liked us, so when you think about it, it is not surprising that I won. I felt honored, not because I was a good cook, but because they liked us so much. The next year, we won the "long term resident" title.

There was a period during that next summer that I met another very nice American. I would go over to visit her at her hotel, the Holiday Inn, and we would swim in the pool. Before we went to the pool we would watch the news on television about the 21 hostages who had been vacationing at a Malaysian diving resort on April 23, 2000, when Muslim extremists abducted them. For weeks we watched daily, hoping to see that they were released. We were so thankful that it wasn't us. I think both of us felt safer living on the small island of Batam.

She was in Batam for about six weeks with her husband, which wasn't enough time for me. Later, when I was back in America I found her again on Facebook.

Most of my vacations during my two-year stay in Indonesia were spent in the United States seeing my children. David and I did take a vacation together to Cairns, Australia, in Queensland. The highlight of that trip was seeing The Great Barrier Reef. One thing that meant a lot to me in Cairns, after I had been in Batam for two years, was just sitting on a bench alone, with no one bothering me. I enjoyed watching the birds, while David went into a drugstore to get us a snack. Life in Indonesia was so different: I couldn't walk alone to a store without men snickering at me, because I was a woman walking alone in a Muslim country. The feel of freedom was so fantastic!

We left Batam early in March 2001. Then for the month of June we went back to Bogor, Indonesia, for extra work that needed to be done. David told me he didn't feel that well, so we were in no way eager to extend our stay. After we left at the end of June 2001, we never returned to Indonesia.

Coming home to Sunnyvale, California, I saw a vase on the living room end table that was full of roses. I thought how nice it was that my son was thinking of me, only I found out later that the flowers were not for me, they were for his girlfriend.

My Caring Friends

Two months ago I sent out e-mail to my friends, asking them if they could please share their weight loss stories with me. For anonymity, all the names have been changed. They have agreed to let me share their letters with you.

Hi Kirsten,
My own overeating downfall is an inconsistent work schedule. I work what is essentially a swing shift, since many of my piano students are of school age, and I feel reluctant to consume a full meal inside my relatively tiny studio while I teach. I had tried to schedule a half-hour of eating time around 6 or 6:30 every night, but my students have appreciated a certain amount of flexibility in my studio scheduling (many of my younger students also participate in athletics, forensics, student council, music ensembles, and some even have after-school jobs), so, more often than not, I had found myself "not having eaten" in nine hours, and, predictably, I'd be ravenous at 9 pm and I ate whatever I could find. But for several months I've been bringing Pure Protein bars and a 16-oz thermos of water to the studio (250 calories each, one at 6 pm sharp, plus a big draft of water between students), and although I'm not crazy about the bars' taste, this seems to be a convenient stopgap measure; it doesn't seem as bulky or intrusive (or noisy) as a sandwich or a piece of fruit, and I'm not quite so hungry after a night of teaching.
My sister offers the following hint she learned in a weight-loss class:

"Never eat when you're overly...
....H ungry,
....A ngry,
....L onely,
....T ired, or
....S tressed."
Rebecca

Hi Kirsten,
I am realizing that I don't have a lot of vivid memories about my weight loss attempts. I do remember going to a University of Maryland Outreach program one evening which inspired me to lose weight when I was in my 30s. One thing I really remember is that the speaker said that your stomach feels full about twenty minutes after you eat, so that if you eat slowly, you will feel full and have eaten less than someone who gulps down their food. I feel like it's lucky that I am a slow eater! I think that I started doing a food diary at that time and kept a calorie count of everything I ate. I did lose a lot of weight that time, but my stomach always still seemed to be as big as ever! Finally I just decided to stop dieting. I did ok for a while, but gradually gained that weight back and more. I think that stress and lots of responsibilities did me in (along with just liking to eat the wrong thing!) I know that I tried to cut back at various other times, but the details are vague in my mind.

Take care, and love to everybody,
Maria

Dear Kirsten,
In a nutshell: Two years ago, I lost 60 pounds (starting weight of 190) by going on a medically-supervised very low calorie meal replacement program, i.e., a fast. I have gained back about 5 pounds and am finding weight management to be a real and constant struggle. I still attend a weekly class at the weight management center. Until age 40 (when I gave birth to my son), I was never overweight. I am now 61 years old.
I think that you will be able to judge from that brief synopsis whether I fit the subset of persons in whom you are interested.
With best regards,
Tammy

Hi Kirsten,
I can definitely relate to your experiences. I agree most people don't understand what it's like having to deal with weight issues. They think that our weight or control over food is simply a matter of "willpower", but I know for a fact that it's not. There's a lot of literature out there to suggest that there are deeper physiological processes at work, which make it extremely difficult for some of us to keep away from certain foods, stick to healthy eating habits, or lose pounds as easily as the

average person. I guess the good news is that even these things can be overcome, and we can find we can actually live without a lot of the things we've grown so used to living with our whole life.

For example, when I was growing up with Bob, we used to drink lots of sodas (e.g. Coke, Sprite) in school. That surely led to a lot of my weight gain. I thought I would never be able to stop drinking pop. It must have been some time in college, I had decided to stop drinking pop. At first it was hard; I think I weaned myself off by drinking slightly less sweetened drinks, like iced tea. Then, one day I remember I was at a party or dinner with friends, and was given the opportunity to have some Coke. I tried it -- and was completely disgusted by how sweet it was! It's amazing how that happened. Our bodies & taste buds get used to certain foods, but in the same way they can get "un-used" to them. I'm still trying to break my habits with other kinds of foods (like carbs), but my past experience tells me since I've done it before, I can do it again.

Most importantly, you should realize you aren't alone. There are actually a lot of people out there sharing similar experiences, as I'm sure you're finding in researching your book. I have a particular problem controlling my eating late at night -- I guess I use food as a

way to de-stress from life after work and so on. Most of my calories are consumed late at night, well after dinner. At first I thought I must be crazy, but lo and behold there are actually lots of people who do the same thing! I actually found a Yahoo email group a couple years ago called "Nightgrazers" where people share their experiences. I feel it has helped tremendously in not only sharing ideas about how to deal with the issues, but just knowing I'm not alone out there. So, if you ever feel that you are I'd encourage you to seek out support groups because I can guarantee you that while most people just don't understand what we go through, there is a group of people out there who certainly do.
Sam

Hi Kirsten,
As I mentioned, when I was a kid, nobody made value judgments about people who were overweight. We just commented that it was their “glands" and never really talked about it.

Nobody in my family had any weight problems that I can recall. My Dad went from medium build to what they called “portly" in his 60s -- but later on became quite thin as he reached his 70s and 80s.

One of my grandmothers was what people might call "obese" -- but in those days, she was just referred to as a "big" woman. I have a friend I tend to think of as also a "big" woman. She's probably over 300 pounds and inactive because of health problems and the fact that she was in an accident when her defective Toyota accelerated and hit a pole.

When I see overweight kids I feel sorry for them because of the health problems they face. If I saw them stuffing themselves with junk foods, my first thought might be that they're foolishly making a big health mistake.
From time to time I used to watch the Dr. Oz TV show and he had a lot of programs about obesity. They made me realize that overeating is sometimes triggered by psychological reasons and not just a lack of will power. I know that there's one genetic trigger to grossly overweight people -- but I can't recall what the condition is called.

I try not to judge overweight people as lacking will power -- especially when I see how hard some of the women at the gym work out in the pool and on the machines. Somehow or other I can "tolerate" overweight conditions in women rather than in men. When I see man whose belly hangs way over his body I tend to think of him as lacking self-control. Even though Intellectually I know that the

overweight condition can be due to reasons beyond the person's control.
Lily

Hi Kirsten,
Is your diet counselor able to provide you with extra reading material, or to recommend any? I'm thinking now about "labels." Maybe on Wikipedia or on certain websites if you Google "reading nutritional information" you'll find lots of sources. That's one of the first things my diabetes counselor told me. …

Something else: "Most of us are dehydrated most of the time. We think we're doing ourselves a favor by not having to run to the bathroom every hour, but we're wearing our insides to death by not replenishing liquid," said another counselor at the place I got "trained" in diabetes control. "How is the sugar inside you going to go away if you don't help it along?" And it can be done carefully. Don't glug a gallon of water in ten minutes, that's how stupid people kill themselves. No, drink a half gallon of water over the course of a day. …
Rebecca

This letter is really helpful to me, as I am also a diabetic. I like the part about flushing the sugar along its way with water.

Another comment came from Rebecca, who said:

> Hi Kirsten,
> I know a woman, who for years was worried about her weight and ate nothing but candy and drank Diet Coke, now is a raging diabetic who has lost most of her vision (she walks everywhere or uses Dial-A Ride to shop), and still says she'll eat herself into a diabetic coma when she decides she docsn't want to live any more. She is meticulous about her computer and her genealogy research, but her house is filthy and she has alienated most of her family with her self-absorption. My unanswered question of the day: why does she want to live now?
> Love,
> Rebecca

Oh, this is so sad. Overweight people face a struggle all their lives. This book is to help me, as well as all of you, and maybe the thin people who read this will learn to develop more compassion toward us.

My Semi Colon Is the Best

My husband was sick when we returned home from Indonesia at the end of June 2001. Soon after we returned he scheduled several doctor visits. Something was really wrong. In the past he had used an antibiotic that had helped him to recover from his diverticulosis. This time, it no longer worked.

His doctor used good judgment and eliminated the extra lab tests. She sent him straight to the hospital. I knew surgery would most likely be next. I sat in the waiting room after saying goodbye to him, telling him that I would be there to see him in the recovery room. Then I walked down the hall, entered the waiting area, sat down and immediately started to cry. I was feeling sad for both of us.

About 15 minutes later my children came and I pulled myself together. They waited with me for what seemed like hours. All of a sudden the door opened and the doctor walked out. He walked directly toward me to tell me that my husband was doing fine, and that he was awake in the recovery room. Oh, what a relief. The pressure was building up in me, and when I heard the good news, the valve was turned and the excess steam was released in just a few seconds. After all of us got to see him and talked to him with our cheerful good wishes, my daughter came out of the room and started to cry. I asked her what was wrong and she said, "My Daddy looks old." After surgery no one looks his best, *and even though we all know this, seeing her father so pale was a shock to her.*

Diverticulosis is the inflammation of small pouches along the wall of the colon. Many people have few or no symptoms, but my husband had some abdominal cramping. The damage to my husband was more severe than we had thought. Actually, it was more severe than the surgeon had thought. Half his colon had to be removed. David joked with us saying that he was now a "semi colon."

September 11, 2001

David was home recovering in August and September, during the time we were having our kitchen remodeled. One morning in September, the two workmen who were doing the job came in our house, and immediately asked if they could watch television with us. This would have been an unusual request, but not on this day. We had the television on a half hour before they came and saw the first shocking scenes from the 9/11 attacks of the Twin Towers in New York City.

On September 11, 2001, 19 Al Qaeda terrorists hijacked four commercial passenger jet liners. The hijackers purposefully crashed into the Twin Towers of the World Trade Center, killing everyone in the planes and many others in the buildings. Both towers collapsed within two hours. A third plane hit the Pentagon. The fourth plane crashed on a field in Pennsylvania. The hijackers were heading toward Washington, D.C., but because of cell phones, some of the passengers on this flight had heard about the Twin Towers crash, so they attempted to retake control of the plane. This ultimately caused the plane to crash over a field in Pennsylvania. All the people on all the flights died. Three thousand victims lost their lives. Over 800 firefighters and police died. Almost 200 people were killed at the Pentagon.

As we sat there watching television with the workmen, none of us could believe it. For days and months this terrible event shook America to the core. Here we were, the majestic world leader, and now in just a matter of a couple of hours we all felt much more vulnerable.

For months, friends I e-mailed told me they couldn't understand how this had happened to our country. I had no answer for them. I was thinking the same thing. Was it errors in judgment in our foreign policy, or just fanatics with a mission to uphold? How did the families that lost loved ones cope? I've often wondered about them. One minute life is okay and the next, life is over. I am not sure how people can ever recover from that. We saw the photos over and over on the news channels, terrifying us even more. Soon security was increased at airports and this told the average American that there really was something to worry about.

Solidarity around the globe grew for our country. On September 12, 2001, the French newspaper *Le Monde* said, "Today, we are all Americans." German chancellor Gerhard Schroeder declared Germany's unlimited solidarity with the United States. China, Iran and Cuba also sent their condolences.

The Optimism of Spring

Time passed and spring finally arrived. David and I took a class on landscaping to figure out what to do with our backyard. We asked our neighbor, who had a beautiful garden arrangement in her front yard, to give us her landscaper's name. We had a large area in the backyard that had a circle of sand where an above-ground swimming pool had once stood. We hired our neighbor's gardener and quickly this landscape artist transformed our backyard.

Both my son and daughter were doing well in their jobs and my husband had retired. Neither one of us had wanted him to work longer than he had to. One friend, whose husband was an airplane mechanic, worked until he was 70, and then he told his wife he just couldn't work anymore. He had always done a lot of work around his house, but one day shortly after he retired he was digging up a fence post and hurt his back. The first week he was in a wheelchair, then dementia set in and his life was effectively over. A month later he died. He only had four months of retirement. That is not what David wanted.

Helping Where the Hurt Is – Hurricane Katrina

On August 29, 2005, another crisis hit America. It wasn't politics this time; it was weather. Strong winds headed to New Orleans, Louisiana. There was a tidal surge as a category three hurricane whipped our southern coast. People's homes were ruined, with 80 percent of New Orleans being flooded. Levees broke, which was the cause of the flooding.

Help came too late for many people. Some people waited it out on rooftops or in trees. Evacuation centers almost turned into prisoner of war camps because of overcrowding. I saw all these pictures on television. It really was difficult to see. I saw a diabetic who couldn't get medicine. Some people were not getting enough to eat. The bathroom situation was a disaster because there were not enough bathrooms for the 15,000 to 20,000 people that were in the Superdome. President George W. Bush was told about the severity of the storm. Many people, including me, could not understand why help arrived so late, days and days after it was really needed. Why? Why were these people treated so badly?

I have a keepsake of this event. The book is called, *IT TAKES A NATION – How Strangers Became Family in the Wake of Hurricane Katrina*, edited by Laura Dawn. As I sat in my living room reading it, I noticed that some little sparrows were seeking refuge in the holly bush on the outside of my window. I have a warm feeling inside when I see that these little birds can escape the constant rain of the day. I have this same feeling when I read the stories in Laura Dawn's book.

On page 20 the author talks about Tobi Hawley, who lives in Arizona and is a mother like Kayantae Synigal-Battle who was rescued from New Orleans. Kayantae was close to giving birth when the hurricane hit. She pleaded to go to the hospital. They sent her to a shelter instead. She pleaded a second time with someone from the Red Cross to help her get to the hospital, only to be sent back to a shelter again. FEMA provided her family a hotel room for a few days and then they were on their own.

When Kayantae was at the shelter, she told the interviewers that 5,000 people were there, using only one shower room with eight showerheads. I read that there were many more people there. The point is that there were thousands of people packed in the Superdome. Conditions were terrible. I felt sad for these people.

Tobi, the host mother, went to HurricaneHousing.org to see how she could help, as she had a winter rental that wasn't being used. There were supposed to be free flights for the evacuees, but Continental Airlines told her to call the Red Cross who told her to call FEMA, who told her to call the Red Cross.

This made me sick when I read about it. Why did the airline that has money, hoard it during this disaster? The Katrina victims had mountains before them that would stack up to heaven. The people that really helped them were just other middle class people. I wrote these pages to commemorate the love they gave to help the victims conquer their mountains.

The Miracle of Love

Tobi went to her church and the members of the church agreed to pay the family's airfare. Kayantae was still pregnant on the flight to Arizona. Tobi's OB/GYN doctor offered his services for free to help Kayantae. At the routine first visit, Kayantae had to be flown in a helicopter to the hospital to give birth. The baby was named Amira, after a miracle.

Story after story fills this book. It is such a "feel good" book. Another lady in Texas, Lynn

Viejobueno, (P. 94) hosted the Briant family. The young boy in the family told his mother with glee that the host lady "Has two dogs and a bird!" What excitement, coming from a boy whose family had been through so much. The family decided to move to Texas as it was better than living out of their car.

FEMA gave everyone a flat $2,000, whether they were one person or a family of five. Lynn helped them get $75 worth of vouchers for clothes. The local food pantry gave the family bags and bags of groceries. The local fire chief gave them a gift card from Wal-Mart worth $300. Patrice, the mother, was so happy that she met Lynn.

In California a couple of years ago, after an earthquake struck, we offered to house one of the schoolteachers who lived in the affected area, but he didn't take up our offer. I think he had other friends or relatives who could help him. There is a Yiddish proverb that says, "God loves the poor, but helps the rich." It needs to be modified to say, "God loves the poor, but helps the rich and the middle class picks up the slack."

Fatty Liver Discovery

This first decade of the new century was turning out to be an unsettling time for all of us. There were no catastrophic events in our lives, like the things that happened to the other people I mentioned.

During our kitchen enlargement project, Walter would come over and give some suggestions on how he thought it should be done. Also, he would tell us over and over about how he had lost weight at the Duke Diet Center. I have no doubt that they offered a good program, but he would constantly push his agenda on us.

The problem with Walter was that he just didn't stop. Once he came over to my house, opened the refrigerator door, and threw out the mayonnaise, ranch dressing and other items he deemed were unhealthy. When he left, I just pulled all these items out of the trash and put them back in my refrigerator.

He was really big on vinegar and oil, and once brought over some bread to dip in this mixture. I admit it didn't taste bad, but after eating too much of it, I went to the hospital emergency room at midnight, after suffering four hours of chest pains. The ER diagnosed my problem as "fatty liver." Later, Walter couldn't seem to understand why I would have this reaction, as these foods were so "healthy" to him.

On subsequent visits he continued his Duke Diet Center praise. He kept pressuring me to go to North Carolina for the program. One thing I learned from this experience, which had nothing to do with diet, is that it's just plain rude to visit someone and pester them to follow the diet that you did. After a while I lost interest in seeing Walter. Our visits with him just died down and we lived our separate lives.

My Dark Bloody Mountain

I remember it was in the winter when I had a terrifying experience. My blood pressure had dropped too low, but I didn't know it at the time. While waking up early in the morning to urinate, I fell back into bed and was too weak to get up. David got up to see what was the matter with me. He could tell something was seriously wrong, so he called 911.

I remember strange men talking to me, who told me they were the ambulance crew and they were going to wrap me in a large piece of plastic to take me to the hospital. That was the only time I left my house in a horizontal position, feeling the early dawn air on my face.

I can't remember what procedures they did on me at the hospital until toward the end of my stay, just before being discharged, when I was in a regular hospital room. I noticed that I had started bleeding rectally, but I thought it was a tear from the catheter. The nurse said it wasn't so, then she shrugged her shoulders and said it was hemorrhoids. The floor was dotted with ketchup colored dots the size of small pancakes. This was not just a little hemorrhoid blood. She scolded me as she told me she wasn't paid to be a maid, but she was smiling when she saw David.

I wanted to go home, to get away from this nurse. The doctor decided to take me off nortriptyline, which I was taking for leg pain. He said it had pushed my blood pressure too low, and he gave me another medication for the nerve pain in my leg.

After being home for several hours and noticing that the rectal bleeding wasn't improving, I started wearing sanitary pads. As it got worse I just changed pads more often. My daughter-in-law talked to me on the phone and told me that any bleeding could be serious, so I went back to the emergency room. Three times over the next twelve hours I visited the emergency room, only to be sent home each time after being told, "Honey, you haven't lost enough blood yet."

I was getting weaker. As I walked out of the hospital, I knew I left a trail of blood on the floor, as I could feel it gushing out of me.

David was there to help me. When I saw him, I was sure I saw a smirk on his face as he was talking to another man in the waiting room, telling him this was the third time he had brought me in. You would have to know my husband to know how untrue this twisted thought of mine was. I was having trouble judging situations correctly. He has always been a very loving husband to me, and has never had a smirk on his face when talking about me.

Driving home I sat on a plastic trash bag. Just a couple of nights before I had my 911 visit for low blood pressure, I had colored my hair, as periodically I did this to keep up with the grays, because I like to look attractive. This is my evidence that I was of sound mind and body just days before my darkest hour.

Stepping Into Mental Hell

I was overtired when we got home from the hospital. More than 24 hours had passed with no sleep, as going in and out of the ER during the night does not make a restful night. I was upset and figured I was going to die anyway from the continuous loss of blood. I vaguely remembered a story about a woman who had walked to the freeway to take her life. I was thinking, because of the smirk I thought I saw on my husband's face that he didn't love me anymore. I was so mixed up that I started walking down the street while thinking about the lady who walked to the freeway and took her own life. I was confused. I thought it was 8:00 p.m. Later I was told that it was 4:00 a.m. I banged on a neighbor's door, crying and saying that I couldn't go through with it, that I could not take my own life.

My friends didn't know what to do with me and called 911 to get help. The police came and that is where my terror began. I asked if I could just go home, and they wouldn't let me. My husband was there, but that didn't matter. I had to cooperate; otherwise they said they would use force. They stuck me in a patrol car. When I asked for a dollar to make phone calls they responded to me as if I was a bag of groceries in the backseat.

I didn't know where I was going. I was very weak, as I was still bleeding. I have no memory of how I walked out of the police car into the county hospital. I spent about 12 hours there calling everyone, my husband, my son, and my daughter, over and over to have someone get me a lawyer as I was being held against my will. They took away my shoes, and even took a shoelace string from my blouse. It was only about two hours until the sun came up, and I was amazed at what a short night it had been.

When I got up to make another phone call on the free phone, I noticed some people eating. One nice lady said to me, "Honey, would you like some?" I had three meatballs and a small container of milk. I sat there for hours between the drunks and the crazies. One woman shouted obscenities as she hurled her milk carton across the room. One man stood up and started a fistfight with a guard. I was exhausted, but couldn't fall asleep for one minute because I was so afraid.

There were rooms off to the side of this circular room where people were in the dark, but I saw guards flipping on and off what looked like a light switch just outside these rooms. I was afraid; what was happening in these rooms? My son and daughter-in-law came to see me early in the afternoon, and I was escorted out to talk to them for five minutes.

After what seemed like an eternity, with just one five-minute break, I had a short interview by a professional, who deemed I was not well. Late in the afternoon two men approached me and said my name. They were the ambulance drivers who said they had come to take me to another location. I felt so wonderful and safe in the back of that ambulance for the 45 minute drive to the new facility. More than anything, I felt SAFE and so good that I was no longer at the county hospital where the policeman had brought me. Months later I received a bill for $1,700 for that 12 hour stay, which included no medical care, and only three meatballs and a carton of milk.

I can't remember how I came to be sitting in a chair being interviewed by another doctor. By this time I had gone more than 62 hours without sleep. All I can remember was that they handed me the phone and I heard my daughter's voice say, "Mom, don't worry, these people will take good care of you." I clung on to that thought. Before the doctor spoke to me I had to sign some paperwork, and all I could think of, as these were questions of financial responsibility and my insurance coverage, is that these people were going to try to have me sign a statement so that they could take all our money away. I was very confused. I had lost too much blood and I had not slept for more than 60 hours. After the interview I was given a pill, went to bed, but didn't close the door to the room, because I was afraid they would lock me in. I slept for a few hours, but was awake at 4:00 a.m. I walked down the hall, but was told to go back to bed.

Once it was daylight I looked around and I could see there were bars on the window of my room. Outside there was a large redwood tree. This tree became my tree of hope. We were told to attend classes. This prison had three meals a day. I learned to be friendly to the guards and the nurses; otherwise they might not be friendly back. There was one male nurse who liked me. Another nurse threatened me with insulin if I didn't get my blood sugar numbers down. I had no control over my diet, and we had no exercise. We were not allowed outside, so I never got any fresh air. How was I going to get my blood sugar numbers down?

Blood, Fresh Air and Rain

The doctor who first saw me as I entered the second facility said he thought I had lost a lot of blood by the way I was sitting in the chair. Midway through the week I was told I needed a blood transfusion. I was escorted upstairs to the third floor half an hour before midnight. The nurses on the third floor were very nice to me. As I lay there during the night, I could feel the cool breeze coming in through the window that was slightly open. This wonderful feeling of fresh air is a feeling that most people don't miss until they don't have it anymore. Hearing the constant gentle rain rocked me to sleep.

There was another inmate at facility #2 who had been there longer than I, and she showed me the ropes. When you are incarcerated you need to associate yourself with the strong ones of the group, not the weak. Twice there were fire drills, but we never were let out. Once, there was a real kitchen fire on the floor below us. My new lady friend said to me, as we walked around looking for ways to escape a fire if we had to, "I don't know what we are all worried about, just one week ago, we wanted to kill ourselves anyway."

At the end of a week, before leaving facility #2, I had to sign a paper stating that I would take additional classes and commit myself to additional evaluation. These classes lasted from two to three weeks, and it was at their discretion as to when I would be released. I was also informed that if I didn't sign this paper, the facility would not release me. There was not much choice available to me. It was either stay at facility #2 until who knows when, or sign their paper.

At my exit interview from facility #2, I also had to sign a paper acknowledging that I could not purchase a gun for five years after my discharge. Little did they know that just a month after leaving the #2 facility, I was at a garage sale where a man was selling foot-long hunting knives, and I could have purchased any of them without a permit.

As I walked out of facility #2, I could feel the fresh air on my face again. The hospital had valet parking, and the parking assistants were dressed all in black. To me, these parking attendants looked like the guards from the county hospital. I panicked, shoving my husband into the car so that we could get away quickly. I was afraid they might take us both back to the basement.

Tea Party Joy

Upon leaving the hospital, I asked David to take me to a fast food restaurant to get a large coke. Then we drove straight to see my granddaughter. She had been told that I had hurt my back and that is why I didn't visit her. What joy I had in playing tea party with her, as I sat on the floor with her and nine stuffed animals. She didn't treat me any differently than a week before. She poured me imaginary tea in a small pink cup. Maybe the tea wasn't real, but the freedom was.

Following my stay at the second hospital I checked the scale and could not believe it. I had lost 12 pounds in one week. That is too much weight to lose in one week.

For two to three weeks I had to go to outpatient classes, and only got Tuesday and Thursday off, because I pushed really hard to get a few days off to go swimming. Since exercise is valued so much in the mental health mindset, I was given these two days off each week. I remember the first time I went back and sat on the locker room bench, I felt my secret was hidden from the others, but the main feeling I had was that I was just as "free" as they were, even though my freedom was only on Tuesday and Thursday. I never admitted the truth to the other people in the gym about what really happened to me. Some of them may find out by reading this book.

At facility #3 I met two familiar faces that I had seen at facility #2. One came a few days after I had started outpatient classes. He told me that during noon visiting hours, one of the patients walked out of the facility while visitors were walking in. After visiting hours they did the head count, as they did three times a day, and the nurses came up one number short. This caused a real frenzy to the mental health staff. For hours they searched every area, looking in all the closets, behind all the corners and under the beds but he couldn't be found. During the seven o'clock visiting hours after dinner, he walked back in with the other visitors. Of course, he wasn't wearing any shoes, like the rest of us, but perhaps he just wanted to get a little fresh air.

Once I had regained my strength from the blood loss, and I had been attending facility #3 for two weeks, I told the psychiatrist that I felt I didn't need the classes anymore. Their medication for depression didn't work on me. I had to cut the dose in half, and then half again, as it was making me shake like a washing machine agitator. The psychiatrist said, "Kirsten, I don't believe you are depressed." I never was depressed. I lost too much blood, which was the problem. One doctor said I had a "loss of oxygen to the brain."

One thing I learned from this experience. Never, ever, say to anyone that you are thinking of taking your own life. You can talk to strangers about the details of your sex life, or your financial life, but never mention your thoughts of suicide. My situation, which was misdiagnosed, was due to a rapid blood loss and lack of sleep. I've done nothing shameful to be embarrassed about, but because of the stigma of being in a mental health hospital, I felt hesitant to talk to others about what happened to me.

Weeks later, after I was finally discharged from all three facilities, I saw my regular doctor. She reviewed my medical notes and said that she thought I had diverticular disease, which had caused the massive bleeding.

A Man without a Wife Is Like a Vase without Flowers
–African Proverb

David and I talked about this heading after I told him I wanted to use it. Then he suggested an alternative. He said I could use, "A man without a wife is like a fish without a bicycle." He is such a wonderful man to love!

Starting the beginning of 2008 we began planning and getting excited about my daughter's upcoming wedding, at Cornerstone Gardens in Sonoma, California. Several times prior to the wedding David and I went there to take measurements, draw a diagram of the barn, and record where all the outlets were for lighting. It was to be a grand affair, a wedding all would remember as special. In February we went to the fabric store, where my daughter picked out cranberry colored organza and we ordered 20 yards, for me to make a flowing canopy to hang from the ceiling. This was to hang over a royal throne for my beautiful queen and her groom to sit on when they weren't dancing.

After visiting several bridal shops, my daughter found the perfect wedding dress. I kept searching and searching for the right dress for myself, as I have only one daughter and I wanted to look good for her. A friend from my gym worked with me when I brought over my dark royal blue mother-of-the-bride dress, to match the colors for the crystal necklace that she designed and made for me. At the wedding, several women complimented me on the necklace. One woman did it three times, and I got the feeling that she really wanted my necklace. At that point I knew my friend had created a masterpiece.

The previous January I began to lose weight, and was down to 180 pounds by the time of the October wedding. Unfortunately, after the wedding, I resumed my old eating habits and regained the weight I had lost. This was not the first time I had regained lost weight.

During the wedding, the family, parents, in-laws and other relatives stayed at a rented ranch house within walking distance of the wedding venue. On our last day there, my sister-in-law cooked us a magnificent breakfast with eggs, bacon, toast and tea. As we all sat around a long table recalling our recent wedding memories of just days ago, I remembered thinking how nice it would be if we had a reunion and did this again next year. But I knew this would never happen, since the relatives had come from Arizona, Georgia, Hawaii and Chicago. Some things in life only happen once.

The wedding party, which included the maid of honor and the groomsmen as well as the bride and groom, stayed at a furnished mansion a couple of miles away. Plenty of parties took place at this mansion during the days around the wedding, and there was always an overabundance of food. Every time I visited, snack food was sitting out on the kitchen counter.

Flying in from Hawaii were the groom's parents. Flying in from New York were the groom's siblings. Our side of the family had guests coming from Arizona, Georgia and Maryland. I didn't know it at the time, but the relative from Georgia has since become a very good friend of mine.

The groom's parents brought several Hawaiian leis with them. The groom's sister performed a Hawaiian chant for the wedding. The bride's best friend recited a special poem. She is the same friend that had met us in New York for the PR Student of the Year Awards. My three-year old granddaughter, who wore a white dress and a red sweater, was the flower girl. The groom's little nephew, dressed in a black suit, was the ring bearer. My little grandson, just conceived weeks before, was hiding under my daughter-in-law's red dress.

A week later, David and I flew to Oahu, Hawaii to attend a luau to celebrate their wedding, as many of the groom's Hawaiian friends were not able to make the trip to

California. This way, my daughter and new son-in-law got to visit Hawaii again. Even though these strangers at the luau didn't know us, they were very nice to us, as if they were our friends. Rows of tables were set up for the feast, and there was one round table that had two white frosted cakes that said Congratulations, J & J, 10-10-08. It was definitely an affair to remember.

Winning Is Wonderful!

Whether I win an award in the weight loss class or not, I am still a winner, as I have lost 26 pounds so far. This is just the beginning. To walk a mile, you go step by step. Translated to weight loss, that means you lose one pound first, then the next, and then the next. You just chip, chip, chip away at it.

Dear Maria,
The awards were given out today. I didn't get first, I didn't get second, but I did get third. It was by percentage of weight lost. My prize is a $25 gift card at Whole Foods. To me it means everything. I knew Irving would beat me. He had a 12.6% loss, but what I didn't know is that another lady, in the other class, lost 14.7% of her weight, so she got first place, the $100 gift card or a trainer. Irving was offered the choice too, but took the $50 Whole Foods card. They just handed me the $25 card, as they know that I only go to water exercises and walk. I was recognized in being the most consistent of them all in that I had lost weight every week. It sounds immature, but I am so happy that I won a prize.
You had asked me to tell you what happened, and because you have given me so much support and love, I wanted to write to you immediately.
Your friend, Kirsten
P.S. I think I forgot to tell you that my weight loss was 11.8%.

Dear Kirsten,
I'm so happy for you! That is really wonderful! Bask in your success and the recognition for all of your hard work and great attitude. You are doing so great! That's wonderful that you were also recognized as being the most consistent. I wish I could give you a big hug!! Enjoy your $25 Whole Foods gift card. There are so many great choices there. You will have a treat picking out what you can get for your prize!
Take care, and thanks for letting me know! You made my day!!!
love and congratulations to you, Maria

Hi Kirsten,
Congratulations on your weight loss of 26 lbs! That is a fantastic achievement. I know what you mean about how hard it is -- but I also know how good that feels to lose that much weight, and how totally "worth it" it is. Lately, I've been struggling slightly with my weight -- I have gained about 6-7 pounds in the last month. I attribute it mainly due to work-related stress and general anxiety about these difficult times. But hearing your story inspires me.
Thanks for sharing, and keep up the great work!
Sam

Sixteen people came to the weight loss awards ceremony. Most were from the other class. One nice word came from one of the pencils as I left the class. She said, "You have been remarkably successful." Irving said, "The two of us can go shopping together, and buy all the 'bad stuff' at Whole Foods." I have seen some delicious looking cakes and large chunks of chocolate at that store, but I shall leave this for other customers to purchase.

This morning when I checked my fasting blood sugar reading it was 99. That is my First Prize. This new lifestyle is turning out to be a win-win for me.

Tip # 14
"To Lengthen Thy Life,
Lessen Thy Meals."
–Benjamin Franklin

This is an area I want to cover, as there are studies that claim eating fewer calories can lead to a longer life.

Longevity in Animals

Some scientists say that it is your genetic make-up that determines how long you live. A scientist named Thomas E. Johnson studied a set of vital genes that he calls "geronto-genes." Other scientists call these genes "longevity determinant genes." Still other scientists think that it is 7,000 genes that control aging, not just a few.

Sixty years ago, Dr. Clive M. McCay, from Cornell University, extended the life of rats by using calorie-restricted diets. Their life span increased by 50 percent. The article said that fewer calories not only extended the rats' life span, but also stabilized the rats' mental functioning and physical fitness.

Next, low calorie experiments were done with fish and guinea pigs. This was also shown to extend their lives. Observed was a delay in the onset of diseases like heart disease, cancer, diabetes and other diseases that often hit older people.

In 1987 tests were started on monkeys by the National Institute on Aging. The University of Wisconsin was also conducting tests. Observations made after 10 years showed the monkeys on the restricted diet were much healthier, more active, and their lab tests for blood pressure and blood sugar levels, as well as cholesterol levels, all improved due to the lower number of calories consumed.

Touching, A Gift Of Love and Life

One point that I noticed about other cultures is that having close family ties contributes to longevity. "Reach out and touch someone" is not just a catchy phrase; it is a therapeutic suggestion to help people. Many cultures instinctively know this.

In 1988 there was a study at Stanford University by neuroscientist Robert Sapolsky and his colleague Michael Meaney from McGill University, where they attempted to prove this theory. They spent 15 minutes a day for three weeks handling newborn lab rats. When the rats were an old age of 28 months, they found that these rats could swim mazes much better than their untouched peers, and they could swim them just as well as younger rats. In the handled rats, a region of their brains had developed extra receptors, which kept their stress hormones down. Rats are not humans, but these scientists recorded a remarkable difference.

Family, Medicine and Sanitation

Leonard Sagan attributes longevity to the increased strength of the family. Two centuries ago, and even in some places today, children were to be seen, and not heard. This is how the affluent people lived, while poor people's children were often more included in the family, even if it was just to help with the chores.

His ideas are controversial because many scientists feel improved sanitation and medical breakthroughs play a large role in life expectancy. No doubt, all these facets do, but it is good to include possible contributing factors.

Be Mindful When Exercising

For all the people that give exercise credit, there are some who point out that if there is a health issue in your family, (i.e. several of your relatives have died early of heart attacks), then family members need to be wary of exercise that taxes the heart. I think this is just common sense.

These naysayers bring up a case of a 50 year old man who was running for exercise, and had a heart attack. I am familiar with injuries that exercise can do to the joints. As a result of exercising, I got plantar fasciitis by walking two hours when I was in my 40s. Also, from doing arm movements too vigorously similar to breast stroke, I developed tennis elbow. I used to exercise a lot in the pool in Indonesia. I suspect that contributed to my frozen shoulder.

The Balance of Maintaining a Healthy Body and Mind

My Aunt Pamela is 88 years old. She told me about one of her relatives that lived to be 97 and he was still ballroom dancing. He had tended the farm, but what is also amazing is that because he wasn't sure if his heirs could handle all the financial aspects of caring for the property, he also kept meticulous records of the expenses of the farm until the day he died.

My Aunt Pamela worked many years in a hospital and just for the fun of it she kept advertisements of the newest medications. She researched those medications years later, to see which ones held to their promises.

At her last doctor visit her doctor told her to take a calcium pill with vitamin D and to take several deep breaths a day. She sort of chuckled a bit about the "deep breaths." She said some days are not so good when you are old, and at these times she remembers what her mother told her, "Just shut out everything and focus on being dumb." I think most people have some of those "dumb days."

Aunt Pamela pointed out that the people in other countries walk much more than Americans. When she visited Europe, after taking public transportation during the last leg of her journey, she walked. She is not into exercising, but she likes to walk. Walking has served her well in the past, so she doesn't see a need to change.

One of her friends, who is over 80, went to the doctor and he told her she needed to get her cholesterol down. When she reported back to the doctor that the pill didn't agree with her, she was surprised when he changed his advice: "There is no reason for you to take it, as you are doing well for your age."

Aunt Pamela said that from her observations many people live the same number of years whether they have a good attitude or a poor attitude toward life. To carry this further she said some people are very positive in the way they fight cancer, while others are very mad. In her opinion, the outcome is often the same. To her, quality of life is the name of the game, not just reaching an older and older age. She doesn't want to live to be 101, celebrating her birthday in a nursing home. With her three children, all of her grandchildren, plus all of her friends and their children, she is very happy. Family, and love of family, which I will talk about later, plays a big part in longevity.

She knows a man who is in his late 80s and whose health is poor. He lives with his family, but due to his poor attitude he works on pulling down the younger members of the family. He wants to die, but just can't seem to do it yet. Aunt Pamela says that when older people are in a controlled situation, either by being in a nursing home, or another type of controlled situation where they are limited, because of their own lack of hearing or vision loss, this makes them become more alone. This can undermine their health.

In closing, Aunt Pamela said she thinks genes have a lot to do with longevity. Her mother lived to be 91. Her sister-in-law lived to be 96. Her brother lived to be 89. My aunt has some good strong genes on her side.

The Age Questionnaire

Many medical experts feel that if you are 20 percent overweight, you should try to lose weight, even if it is only 10 percent.

But there is another idea that as people age, many of them begin to lose weight, and are at risk of becoming frail. The experts that feel this way say that a person does not want to be skin and bones when they get older. This frailty can lead to falls, and the problems of recovering after the fall. For me, that doesn't mean to stop moving and start watching television.

Have you ever taken one of those tests in women's magazines that tell you how old you really are? We all know our chronological age, but we don't know our biological age. Most of these tests cover your medicines, your exercise, your smoking, your sugar and salt intake, and your use of alcohol. Some will even cover health problems, such as heart disease and hypertension. They may ask if anyone in your family has cancer. Some of it reminds me of the forms you are given as a new patient in a doctor's office.

My Mantra, Just Move

There is also another tool for longevity that isn't at the gym. Two older people I know do this type of exercise. You can lose extra calories just by moving. Climb the stairs instead of using the elevator. Vacuuming, lawn mowing and cleaning windows all count. Even mopping floors makes it to the list.

Fun activities count as well. Volleyball, horseback riding, bowling and canoeing all count as exercise. Maybe it doesn't register at the highest number of heart beats per minute, but it all adds up, just like the food on your plate.

A friend of mine told me the only time her husband gains weight is when he can't run, as when recovering from a sports injury. For many of us who are not runners, low impact aerobic exercises might be the best. I really believe there is some exercise out there for everybody.

Bob is Ninety

My father-in-law, Bob, who is 90 years old, gave me an interview. My son-in-law says that Bob will "outlive us all." Bob shared his thoughts on aging with me.

He was born in 1920. In his youth, and for most of his life, he stood six feet tall, but now he has shrunk down to five feet, nine inches. From 2-24-2010 through 3-11-2011 he has recorded his weight every day. He was a maximum of 146.6 pounds on 3-30-2010 and a minimum of 136.0 pounds on 2-12-2011. There is NOTHING wrong with this man's brain. He does give genes a lot of credit for his longevity, and said his father lived to be 96 years old, but he also says part of it is luck.

The Basement Track

He used to go hiking until he reached the age of 89. Then he went walking locally in his neighborhood. Because of the harsh winters where he lives, he has made himself a track in the basement, where he can walk every morning.

His wife passed away two years ago, but he seems to be doing well on his own. I know he must have times of suffering, as I have suffered on and off for 20 years following my mother's death.

He lives in his own home and grills his food; he told me specifically that he doesn't fry it. For breakfast he eats one piece of bacon, one egg and a bowl of high fiber cereal, as well as a small glass of orange juice. Bob said that if he notices that his weight is increasing he cuts back on the calories he consumes.

10,000 Steps Each Day

There was a book that came out at the end of the 1960s by Kenneth H. Cooper, a former Air Force Colonel from Oklahoma. The author stressed 10,000 steps per day. Bob started walking again.

During the 60s, President John F. Kennedy was aware that America's school children were becoming overweight and out of shape. Our country had changed and machines had replaced heavy farm work. Factory jobs had also introduced machines and human labor decreased.

Bob continued: People didn't have to do much for entertainment now that there was television and all they had to do was sit. The world was changing. President Kennedy introduced a new program to help the school children. He felt "The strength of our democracy is no greater than the collective well-being of our people."

In 1963 there was a "Progress Report by the President on Physical Fitness." President Kennedy wanted Americans to return to the physical hardiness of years gone by. No one was chopping firewood anymore, and we all spent evenings watching television.

The Chicken Fat Song

One of Bob's daughters was in grade school at the time, and the "in" thing for physical fitness was to have the children follow along to the instructions of the "Chicken Fat Song." There are two entries on *You-Tube* where you can see this song. On one you can even see some children in a 60s classroom.

Mark Wineka authored an article on the web talking about his "childhood of horrors" in living through the "Chicken Fat Song." He says, "Almost 50 years later, the song still haunts me." Here is a tidbit you won't find written on the Web. The Chicken Fat Song was on a small size 33 rpm record, which resembled the 45 rpm record that ran at a faster speed. At Bob's daughter's class, the teacher thought it was a 45 rpm record to be played at this faster speed, and not a 33 rpm record. Those poor children were moving even faster than the song's original speed. It is no wonder, that many children didn't like it. A lot of grade school children during the early 1960s had trouble forgetting this six minute song, as the schools played it every morning. "Touch downs, push-ups, go go go, and give that chicken fat back to the chicken," are some of the lyrics.

The Betty White Syndrome

I asked Bob what he thought about the idea if he could live to be 120 years old. He didn't like it. He said people are no longer accepting what it is like to be truly old. We are all living in the

"Betty White Syndrome," where 90 is really 60 and we will be able to skydive into our graves. He says the new philosophy is that people should get older without getting old.

There are limitations when you get old, but the media doesn't want to know about them. They only want to hear about very active old people. They don't want to know if you are 90 and have outlived all your money.

Quality of life is very important to Bob. He told me about a woman who was on Medicare whose life was extended by four years by medical procedures, and once she left the hospital she couldn't take care of herself. She had to go to a nursing home where she spent down all her money and thus ran herself into total poverty.

There was an article about this in the New York Times, July 18, 2008 by Anemona Hartocollis. She talked about Hazel Homer who was 99 years old, and would have probably passed away in a year due to her aging heart, but she was given a special pacemaker and defibrillator. Over the next four years this lady, who had only been in the hospital during the birth of her daughter, was hospitalized nearly every other month for heart failure and fluid in her lungs. Those last four years were not very pleasant for her.

The Envelope of Old Age

Susan Jacoby has written a book called *Never Say Die: The Myth and Marketing of the New Old Age*. Her views are different than many, but parallel to what Bob says. She points out that as we age, people's health worsens overtime and their financial resources dwindle. An average person is hard pressed to have enough money to survive a 36 year retirement, but she says that the media tells us if we can't do this, something is wrong with us.

She makes a lot of good points in her book. I can personally attest to her belief that the "boomers," like me, do have this illusion in their thinking that if we can just eat right and exercise, we can put off aging forever. I know this isn't true, but part of me has been programmed to think that I can push the envelope farther and farther down the road so old age may never overtake me.

Bob still thinks genes have a lot to do with longevity. Two of his uncles lived to be in their nineties. He can remember when he took his Uncle Edgar out on his 92nd birthday. He mentioned another aunt who was 91 years old. She was in a nursing home and had some dementia. She told Bob, "I don't know who you are, but I am sure happy you came to see me." Bob is a remarkable man. He publishes a bi-monthly newsletter for his immediate family that usually contains 6,000 to 8,000 words. He talks about what is happening in his life and phone calls he has had from his children. We just received letter number 613.

Family, Friends, Fruits and Vegetables

There is an article in the November 2005 National Geographic, which talks about "The Secrets of Long Life." The author, Dan Buettner circled the globe and focused on three locations, Okinawa, Japan; Sardinia, Italy; and Loma Linda, California. He said that a person's success rate in the longevity game first starts with good genes.

He says it is up to you to establish good habits which may help you live a decade longer. One photo shows a 75 year old man who keeps active by walking most of the day. Another photo shows a 100 year old woman, who just got her driver's license renewed for another five years. Another photo shows an 89 year old Japanese woman squatting while inspecting seaweed. These people all have different stories to tell about their old age.

The summary is that none of the people interviewed smoke, and their families are very important to them. They remain active every day and have a strong social network of friends. They also eat fruits, vegetables and whole grains. I can see this as a beautiful picture, but not the reality of what happens to the majority of people when they get old. Bob, who is 90, set me straight on this. This article is wonderful to wish for, and strive for, but most of us will never be in National Geographic.

The Strength of a Smile

Love is another factor that some experts feel helps with positive aging. When I spoke with a 92 year old man at a senior center, I asked him what keeps him going. He said with a smile, "Breathing and poker."

Here is a quote that comes from Jeanne Calment, who died at 122 years old. "Always keep your smile. That's how I explain my long life."

I smile a lot on the outside when I see people I enjoy being with. Inside I am dead serious about losing this extra weight and never letting it come back.

Yesterday I cut a bouquet of small white flowers from a tree in my backyard. Placing them in a vase, I saw one blossom just dangling in mid-air, hanging from an invisible thread. There was a tiny black spider midway down this invisible thread. I wondered if the spider would be able to hold on to his catch, which was much larger and heavier than he was. But the blossom fell to the table and he wasn't able to do it.

My thoughts turned inward. Am I going to be able to effectively handle my weight loss? Am I going to succeed, and not drop the ball in defeat like the spider? He attempted to do something many times his strength, sort of like my climbing down Mount Everest. But, I will, I will, I will! It is one of the greatest challenges of my life.

Macadamia Macaroons

I woke up a little hungry at five in the morning. I was asleep at 10:00 p.m. the night before, so I wasn't worried about not getting enough sleep. I decided to do something with this morning alertness, so I walked over to the kitchen to straighten up the counter and improve on the cleaning job I had done the night before. On the counter, I flattened out the empty saltine box. On that box I saw a photo of macadamia macaroons. There were six on the plate all drizzled with chocolate. Why is this recipe on a box of crackers?

I tossed the empty box in the trash and opened a new box, to eat just one. For the cruel humor of it I turned the box, and there it was again, the photo of the macadamia macaroons. The alcoholic doesn't have to bring bottles of liquor in his house, but I need to have food in my house. How many times are those cookies going to appear? I'm strong; I will fight; there will be no more turning the box.

Georgia on My Mind

Georgia was supposed to be a new beginning for us. For several years we had looked for a more rural property as a place to live. We wanted something better than the postage stamp size lot we had in the San Francisco Bay Area. The Georgia pines pointed like arrows to the sky, and the comfort of the woods was something that we didn't have living in our suburban California home.

Often, when people retire, they long for a "special" location where they think they will be happy. In April we visited David's cousin in Georgia. From those three weeks we felt we liked the location well enough to consider moving there. The summer vacation of 2009 was the beginning of a long journey.

After arriving in Georgia we traveled from Atlanta to Savannah. David's cousin took us to see the Stately Oaks Plantation near her home. David and I drove to see the pride of the old South, Confederate President Jefferson Davis, General Robert E. Lee and General Stonewall Jackson, all carved on the side of

Stone Mountain. Since I figured that we might never get to see Mount Rushmore, I was happy to see the portraits of these men.

The Taj Mahal

After all the sightseeing, we returned to Stockbridge, Georgia, where I spent many mornings and afternoons sitting on the front porch of our cousin's home. I was so at peace with all the natural beauty around me. The aura I felt was of immeasurable beauty, and thus I named her house the Taj Mahal. No matter which way I turned, I saw green leaves swaying in the breeze. Yellow and white butterflies added splashes of color. Surrounding her house was a botanical garden, without a fence and gate.

I sat in silence on her porch as my soul was touched.

***"See how nature – trees, flowers, grass –
grows in silence;
see the stars, the moon, and the sun, how
they move in silence…
we need silence to be able to touch
souls."
–Mother Teresa of Calcutta***

Don't Let Doubts Destroy Us

We visited Callaway Gardens and saw more beautiful butterflies. Of special interest to me was The Little White House in Warm Springs, Georgia, where Franklin D. Roosevelt came to heal his body that had been wounded by polio. There was a handwritten letter in the museum section of the home that said, "The only limit to our realization of tomorrow will be our doubts of today. Let us move forward with strong and active faith." signed Franklin D. Roosevelt.

This is the third time I have read this quote, and feel that I can apply it to my weight loss journey. Just move on with strong and active faith, and don't let our doubts and fears stop us from our goals. Don't let negative feelings creep up to destroy me just because of a cookie photo on a cracker box. Don't let my lusting for a big fancy breakfast with an omelet and hash browns sabotage the rest of my progress. Don't let my desire for a big high calorie dinner of bratwurst and potatoes, with Lebkuchen for dessert, knock me to the ground.

I have encountered this quote by Franklin D. Roosevelt several times. I interpret it to mean that I should not be timid. Even though we were 60 years old, we should not let doubts stand in our way. We should be brave like the patriotic Americans of the Revolutionary War, who fought for our freedom. People never do anything if they are afraid to take the first step.

After a fun and beautiful three weeks visiting with our relatives, seeing the alligators up close at Okefenokee National Wildlife Refuge, visiting Habitat For Humanity, and visiting Plains, Georgia, the home of President Jimmy Carter, and followed by a lot of discussion between ourselves, David and I decided to make the move from California to Georgia. We needed our car, so we drove the 2,000 miles.

On The Road Traveling East

This is where the fun adventure starts. We had seen Arizona several times before, but this time we were just traveling through. Once we even made it to New Mexico with our daughter. Remembering that we had driven round trip from Sunnyvale, California to Vancouver, British Columbia, in December, facing snow along the way, we took our courage to attempt the 2,000 miles ahead of us.

I had lived in Texas as a child, but had never before driven through the Pan Handle. As we approached Oklahoma, we knew it was a place that neither of us had seen before. We stopped in Oklahoma City. That evening we talked to the hotel clerk to get directions to the memorial to the victims of the Oklahoma City bombing. She said it was close and gave us a map, but we never found the exact location that evening. The next morning we ventured out again, before continuing our journey, and found it.

This memorial was where the bombing took place at the Alfred P. Murrah Federal Building. It has a large reflecting pool and a field of 168 chairs made of bronze and stone, honoring those that died on that terrible day. It was a very moving experience. Looking back, it would have been a gigantic mistake if we had missed this.

Graceland Rocks

Next, we drove through Arkansas and Tennessee, stopping to see Graceland in Memphis, Tennessee, the home of Elvis Presley. After getting our tickets, we walked through the property like a herd of cattle. I had always wanted to see this place. In his home,

Elvis had a long white sofa in the living room, and it was interesting to see the accordion folds in the fabric-covered ceiling of the poolroom. All the furnishings seemed frozen in a 1960 décor to honor the King of Rock and Roll. It was impressive, considering Elvis purchased this house when he was only 21 years old. It was for him and his parents. The next day we drove through Tupelo, Mississippi, the birthplace of Elvis, but did not stop.

We passed through Alabama next, and after six days of travel we were in Georgia. Our cousin helped us by letting us stay with her until we could find a place to live. We knew from our first visit that there were a lot of churches in Georgia, but truthfully I was surprised when the realtor started to quote scripture in the car.

Both David and I had grown up in Maryland and felt we could re-adjust to the summer humidity, but we got our first surprise when we toured the Hay House in Macon, Georgia in August. We didn't see all of the seven levels, including the famous cupola, because it was just too hot. I found myself gravitating more to the rooms that had fans than to the rooms with historical objects.

I Touched the Moon

In September we drove to Florida to see David's aunt and uncle. We combined this with a trip to the Kennedy Space Center. Standing in the large museum hangar, I felt really small looking up at five rocket engines. I even got to touch a piece of the moon. It felt like a granite kitchen countertop. We stayed the night at Jupiter, Florida, near the beach, where we met my daughter and son-in-law. I was so happy to hear her voice on the outside of the motel door; I stumbled around the room like an anxious schoolgirl to meet her first date. I was really missing my children. The next day, the four of us visited the Flagler Museum at Palm Beach. After saying goodbye to them, David and I went on to visit the Everglades.

Alligator Anger Ahead

The Kingston Trio wrote a song called "Everglades." It describes a man running from the law through the Everglades. He has to keep moving. His fate was "If the skeeters don't get him, then the 'gators will." I saw those alligators and they were fat, especially around their bellies. I kept thinking of this song as I moved along with the rest of the tourists to catch a glimpse of them. There were five people ahead of me; I could see the alligators on the ground between the grasses of the swamp. One was lying sideways on top of the other. Then I heard a dog-like growl, and I immediately started to walk backwards, until I was far enough away to turn around and walk even faster. The 'gators didn't get me. I played the song over and over on the rest of the trip, happy to still be sightseeing.

Aside from sightseeing, I thought I would share a little of my daily life. After returning home from Florida we started to mow the lawn. The autumn afternoon sun warmed us, while above our heads it was raining leaves. (Our property had over 200 trees. One day I started counting, and stopped three quarters of the way through at 200.) After we had finished mowing the lawn to remove the leaves, the leaves started raining again, just to show us that nature is the king.

During the month of October we went to Virginia to care for my father-in-law, who was going to have hernia surgery. Every day I would prepare dinner, not knowing from one day to the next what I was going to cook. I'd get up in the morning, grab a cookbook off the shelf, thumb through it and stop at a *random page, to pick a recipe for dinner. It was sort of like throwing darts at a target.*

David and I would go to the grocery store to get the ingredients. Bob liked that, as there was always a surprise for dinner. Little did he know that it was also a surprise to me, only I knew about it eight hours before he did.

Bob's surgery went very well, much better than we all expected. By Halloween we started talking about when we would leave to return to Georgia.

The Balloon Boy

The one strange news item that I saw on television during our stay was about the "balloon boy." On October 15, 2009 a couple allowed a balloon filled with helium to float into the air, claiming their six year old son was inside it. When the balloon finally landed near the Denver airport, the boy was nowhere to be found. People were wondering if the boy had fallen out of the balloon, or what might have happened to him. The boy was finally discovered hiding in the family's garage.

The boy slipped up in a conversation caught by the media, when he said to his parents that he thought this stunt was done for a TV show. The incident was deemed a hoax, and the parents were sentenced to some jail time and a $36,000 fine. The three of us shared some fun time talking about how absurd this whole news story was.

What Would Jesus Think?

Churches dotted the landscape in Georgia just as mosques dotted the landscape in Indonesia. Every block had a church. Even small strip malls had small churches included among the stores. Once I saw a gun shop just two doors down from a "Kingdom" church. Just a store away I saw a "No Loitering" sign. What would Jesus think?

I went to a church service where the pastor spoke for one and a half hours, going past the time I had scheduled for lunch. I am diabetic and this was hard on me as I need to keep a tight schedule with mealtimes. I made a mistake, figuring the service would only be an hour long.

Religion and religious talk seemed to permeate the atmosphere in Georgia. Once at the grocery store, a woman who had seen me at church said to me, not "Hello," but "By the way, come join us for Bible study on Thursday." I invited one lady whom I had met walking to come visit me and she immediately said, "Oh, do you know where (and she said the name of her church) is?" When I said "No," she proceeded to give me directions. She just wanted me to come to her church, not to come visit me.

Church should be how you act, and not a building. It should be a spirit of kindness and love toward others, not just a place where people meet. The feeling I got over and over was that everyone wanted me to come to their church, but didn't really want to get to know me. It was as if they got "mileage points" for bringing in new people. I think it is fine for each person to believe what he wants to believe, but to attempt to make "you" into one of "them" is not fair in friendship. My background is German/Lutheran/Episcopalian and how would it be if I lived my life expecting others to become German/Lutheran/Episcopalian and only those converts would be people that I would associate with?

Two very special people live in Georgia that helped us every step of the way. Even when we bought a storm door from Home Depot, Victor came after work with his truck to haul it home for us. Over the course of a year, David's cousin, Victoria, became a very good friend of mine. Her husband, Victor, is made of gold just as she is. I found that when they went away on small trips, (and we babysat their animals), we were all alone in Georgia.

Swimming and Sketching

We explored the senior centers and found "Clayton Beach." I went to drawing classes and swim classes, while David helped beginning students learn how to use a computer. Everyone was quiet in sketch class, so there wasn't much visiting, and I didn't make any friends in that class. In swim class we were supposed to be quiet for the instruction, so I couldn't talk in that class either. As I really like the "visiting" part of life, I didn't make any friends in these two classes.

We tried more than one senior center, and found that they all offered lunch. Sometimes we ate at the different centers to see what they were like. One thing I noticed was that the white people sat at the tables with other white people and the black people sat at the tables with other black people. Once, a white lady whispered in my ear that she had sold her business to a black person. Things don't seem to have changed. Actually, many of the black ladies were friendlier to me than the white ladies. All of the talk was idle talk, but friendly just the same. We made no lasting friends at the senior centers.

Fate stepped in for me in January when I accompanied David to the training classes for the AARP Tax-Aide Volunteers. During the first couple of classes I would sit outside in the hall by the coffee table. Once, the coffee lady had to leave early at 10:00 a.m., so I told her that I would take over and serve the refreshments during the break. The head of the program noticed me and said I had the qualities to be a good greeter. He asked me if I would come on board. I am happy that I did, because that was where I met my one true Georgia friend, Zelda.

Animal Visitors

Early one morning as I was standing at my kitchen window, looking out over my backyard, I saw an animal coming from the left side of the yard. It was larger than a dog, so I just froze as I watched. Then four more came, for a total of five deer. I stood motionless, afraid to move to get my camera, as I knew that would scare them and they would run away. The largest one froze when she saw me in the window. They ate something from the trees, and stood there for five *minutes or longer. I couldn't turn to see the clock or they would have moved on. I wanted them to stay until they decided to move. It was during the cold bleakness of January that I was treated to this beautiful sight. For days I was happy because I had seen the deer.*

In the spring we once had an eastern box turtle walk 50 feet out from our woods, moving very slowly to our back porch. You could see his trail in the grass, like that of a snail that has left a shiny track of mucus across a sidewalk. David was out in the yard and saved him from an inevitable lawnmower death. He called me, and I was able to get the camera to take photos. Turtles are slow and don't scare that easily, which makes them easy to photograph. He was our "special visitor," now forever on Facebook.

One hot evening after a day of rain, the frogs croaked very loudly. David and I stayed up until 1:00 a.m. to get the recording just right. David recorded it on our computer and then we sent this frog message to our friends via e-mail. Maria's cat's ears perked up as he was sitting on her lap, when she opened up our e-mail. Her cat was looking for the frogs.

Aside from Victoria, no one ever came to visit, except in April, when the woman who I did the AARP Tax-Aide "greeting" with came to visit with her husband. Zelda, my special Georgia friend, was there for me those last three months of my stay.

Drive Thru Tax Service

During the tax season was when Zelda and I met. Once a week we laughed together as we shared our stories. In between this, we signed in people who wanted to have their taxes done. Often there would be waiting times as walk-ins came and the schedule got shuffled. Many people of different backgrounds came to have their taxes done. One lady wore a T-shirt that said "Operation Freedom" with a picture of a cross on it. The words sounded military, but the picture showed religion. One lady just wanted a bunch of forms, but was not interested in getting her taxes done. I was suspicious of her motives and sent her on her way, telling her we didn't have extra forms to give out.

Some people acted in strange ways. One lady told us her dog was sitting in the car, and could we please hurry. I think she thought we were a drive-thru tax service. Another lady was in a big hurry, as she told us she left a pot on the stove, and that she could only spare five minutes.

Early one morning, before anyone had arrived, Zelda and I had gone to the ladies room. A woman who was scheduled to have her taxes done came and sat down in the adjoining lobby. Neither of us saw her walk in and thought she had never arrived. Later, walking out to the lobby, I asked her if I could help her, and she said she had a 9:00 a.m. appointment. It was 9:45, and I realized what a mistake we had made. I immediately pulled her into our little hall office and had her sit down to talk with us. Zelda and I both love to talk. I apologized for what had happened and accepted full responsibility for the mistake. All of the tax preparers were busy on other people's taxes, so this patient lady had to wait even longer. Finally, her turn arrived. She stood up and said, "I'm so happy you 'messed up' and we could all visit together." She wasn't mad at us, in fact, just the opposite, and thus all three of us were happy at the outcome.

There were usually doughnuts or cookies in the tax preparation area, which, unfortunately, I enjoyed. To be at the site at 8:00 a.m. was really hard on me. In my sleepy state of mind, those sweets quickly triggered my brain into action. At that point I wasn't even looking at the scale anymore, so I had no idea what my weight was. I had bought some 3X sweaters, but rationalized that they were more comfortable, not at all thinking that the 2X's had become too tight. It is amazing how you can fool yourself into believing and seeing the world as you wish it.

From January onward we prepared the house for sale. Where we lived, the realtors were not doing open houses, so it was difficult to find a local agent. Victoria had a friend who was a realtor on the north side of Atlanta, very far from our area. She couldn't market our house, but she could, as a friend, give us tips on the best way to present our house. Part of this presentation involves having the house sparkling clean and void of clutter.

After painting and repairing items that needed attention, I made sure that everything was clean and in its proper place. Sunday morning was the only half-day off where I could relax, and not feel forced to be ready at 9:00 a.m., with the pillows fluffed and standing in a slant on the bed. Most everyone was in church and a realtor wouldn't think of bringing someone on Sunday morning. The real estate market was so bad, due to the economic and foreclosure crisis, that we were not able to sell our home. At the end of May, after five months without any offers, we put the house up for rent.

My Georgia Jesus

Here is where the magic continues to happen. Many months before, when driving by a cemetery to go to Home Depot, I noticed a statue of Jesus. The first time I ever saw him, his arms lifted up as if to give me love. Every time I passed after that he was just standing there. In one second he offered me what the preacher failed to offer me in one and a half hours. He became my Georgia Jesus—Giver of Love.

I feel that all religions have their own God, but all call him by different names. Most of the religions that I know about have the element of "love your neighbor" written in their beliefs. You will never see me debunking or badmouthing another religion. I won't join one because that is the "only one" that will lead me to heaven. I believe love can seep through a little crack of a closed religion. I have friends who are Jewish, Buddhist, as well as Christian. They are all going to heaven, not just standing on the outside of the door, not fully participating.

In Georgia, somehow I learned that God and Love is God equals Love, and that is what brought me back to California to my friends and family. While visiting Maryland to see Maria, our realtor phoned to say that a couple from Alaska was interested in renting our house. This is such an unbelievable story, but proof that the concept of God equals Love came through for me. Once back in Georgia we contacted the moving company and the trip back to California began.

On The Road Traveling West

It was a sunny day when the moving van pulled in our driveway in Georgia. They arrived late at 2:15 p.m., and not the usual morning arrival that I had anticipated. Around 5:00 p.m. the movers kept the kitchen door open to move out certain pieces. At 5:30 p.m. I noticed that during the past five minutes I had five mosquito bites on my legs. At this point I excused myself and went out for an early dinner at Burger King, as I was tired of being dinner for the mosquitoes. After a brief stay with Victor and Victoria, we set off on another cross-country drive.

Two evenings before we left, we went to a party for a returning serviceman who was home for a brief stay with his family. Again, I was totally aware that I was overeating. The food was delicious, and in my mind, homemade food tastes the best. For me it is ultimately the hardest to refuse or ration. Even after two days I still felt full with all the party food that I ate, but I did refuel for a brief breakfast at McDonald's before we started driving.

Starting the trip back to California, we passed into Tennessee and got gas in Nashville. We kept a cooler in the car at all times with food for lunch, so we didn't need to drive off the freeway searching for a place to eat, which would have cost us time and reduced the distance traveled each day. Often we just pulled over at highway rest stops and ate there.

Standing by Lincoln

We stopped overnight in Springfield, Illinois. The Lincoln home and museum were something that I wanted to see. We planned the route to include this by traveling on Highway 80 going west, whereas we had traveled on Highway 40 going east to Geor-

gia. At the Lincoln Museum I saw wax statues of the Lincoln family. I posed beside Abraham Lincoln and the rest of his family while David took my picture.

Tip # 15
"Be Sure To Put Your Feet In The Right Place, Then Stand Firm."
–Abraham Lincoln

After a night's rest we were driving through Iowa and had a brief stop in Amana. I photographed a "Guten Tag" sign in one of the stores in this village. Farmlands seemed to cover each side of the highway. Endless blue sky and puffy white clouds were our view in the morning as we left Iowa.

We were following a young man driving a tractor who turned his head to see how far ahead of us he was. He must have noticed I was taking pictures of him. As we pulled off on the side road to get gas, I could see he raised his hand as if to say goodbye to us.

Nebraska also was full of farmland. I remember spending the night at a small town near Omaha. Later, during the next day we stopped at Ogallala, Nebraska to see "Boot Hill," the final resting place for many cowboys, drifters and settlers. The Texas cattle were herded all the way north to Nebraska to the railroad. Many men were buried here who ran afoul of the law. The story goes that many of these men were buried with their boots on, thus the hill was named "Boot Hill." A statue of a cowboy sitting on his horse adorns the top of this hill. I have a photo of the cowboy's face, which shows the exquisite detail of the work done by the artist.

The unmowed grass and weeds helped paint a good picture of the history of the site. From 1874 through 1884 many people were buried here. Women and children were buried here also, as the cemetery was not just for outlaws. It was hard to believe that Indians also roamed the territory as you looked down on the paved streets and contemporary houses below.

We spent the next night in Green River, Wyoming. The motel where we wanted to stay had no vacancy. We found another place on the same interstate exit and stayed there for a night. The lady at the desk told us it was easy to get to the grocery store, but she did not give us good directions. We didn't realize that Smiths grocery store was all the way across town. While we were in a local sandwich shop asking for directions, a nice young lady walked in and said, "Oh, are you going to Smiths? I'm driving right past there on my way home and you can follow me." That was so nice of her. After driving through the town, she pointed to the left where the store was. Then she waved goodbye. We were able to stock up on groceries for the next day's travel. One thing I noticed about Green River, aside from their wonderful hospitality, is that the rock formations near the interstate were exceptionally large. I have photos of a hotel where the formation behind it is twice as tall as the building.

"Rocky Mountain High"
–John Denver

The next stop was the Rocky Mountain National Park in Colorado. The mountains range from 7,000 to 14,000 feet. The fields were full of flowers and water skipped excitedly over rocks in the streams. The cold I felt on my face and arms at the highest elevations in no way hampered the splendor before my eyes of the scenery around me.

On Trail Ridge Road, I found myself having to step back and feel that I was just another pebble in God's creation. I was happy to play my small role; I was so content just standing there. We were now high enough to be at the beginning of the arctic region; I could see where the tree line stopped below us. The layers of life were painted before my eyes. I could have stood there until I froze, enjoying the peace.

Tip # 16
"Adopt the Pace of Nature:
Her Secret is Patience."
–Ralph Waldo Emerson

Descending the mountains, we eventually came close to sea level and saw the Great Salt Lake in Utah. It covers an area of about 1,700 square miles, but that fluctuates because it is shallow and there is the factor of evaporation. Unfortunately, because we were also at sea level, it was impossible for us to get the feel of the size of this great lake.

Even getting out and standing on the car's hood wouldn't have put me high enough to take a good photo. Someone should have been there handing out brochures for helicopter rides you could take at the next stop. I learned that because of its high salt concentration, about 27 percent, people can easily float in it. We wanted to get back to our driving, so I didn't get in the water.

Largest Man Made Excavation

One of the last places we spent time touring was the Bingham Canyon Mine. This majestic piece of artwork lies southwest of Salt Lake City. Another name for it is the Kennecott Copper Mine. The owners claim that it is the largest man-made excavation on earth.

Standing at the visitors' area and looking down, you can't really see that it is 3/4 mile deep, but you can see the circular maze created by the company trucks, and you can almost guess that it is two and a half miles wide.

I saw swirls of tan and rust, and streaks of white from one angle. Turning in another direction, I saw several shades of gray, as a cloud cover had altered this image. I took many photos, as I felt it was not to be forgotten, like a mammoth oil painting.

We were anxious to get home to California after this last stop, so we drove through Nevada. After an overnight stay, we entered California. Again, at the end of our trip, we had someone who was good to us, who let us stay in his house while he lived at his deceased mother's house. Edgar let us stay at his house for two and a half months. In San

Jose, we fixed up the house that we had owned for 30 years. It had been rented, but was now to become our personal residence.

The Towels from Georgia

We arrived in Sunnyvale at Edgar's house the afternoon of July 4, 2010, just about a year after we had left. When I called my son he came over with my granddaughter and brought us some dinner. This house was different, with other furnishings, not at all what my granddaughter had remembered. I explained to her that we were staying at a friend's house. Some of our things had been unpacked from the car; the white with red stripe towels were mine, and I had brought them from Georgia. This way, for the two of us, I could feel like it was my home.

Juan was recommended to us as an excellent contractor, so we hired him to fix up our house. Both bathrooms were redone; some hardwood floor was replaced. A new carpet was installed after the walls were painted baby blue and the ceilings painted white. Neutral was no longer a color for me. That is the "put the hoise up for sale" color, or the "rental house" color, but not a color I would choose for myself.

Garage doors were replaced and minor house flaws were repaired. The house was fumigated, and we finally moved in mid-September. After the inside work was done, it took a whole month to landscape the front yard, because it was overgrown in every direction. Now it's tidy and we have a real lawn. It was hard and took a long time, even though the professionals did all the work.

The furniture placement was carefully thought out prior to moving in, so that moving day would run smoothly. A few months after most of the boxes had been unpacked (except for the "dregs"), we were able to start living. Victoria said that since I had moved twice in a year, I am certified to write a book about it.

Another Slim Jim

At a weight loss group in California I met another "weight greeter." She was not a pencil, but she was a "Slim Jim." I think that the facilitators of these groups think that overweight people do not want to see another overweight person in a leadership role. There should be helpers who are overweight and in the process of losing weight, who extend the hand of friendship and support, not just women of the 110 pound variety. She handed some paperwork to me and other prospective members.

David went with me, and to be honest, we both felt a little depressed after hearing the speaker talk. We both could tell that she was depressed. I actually felt sorry for her. She was thin, but she sure wasn't happy. Each person in the group could stand briefly and say what "weight" matters were on her mind. The time allowed would not have been enough time for me. There was no scale there, and for my purposes, this is a very useful tool to help people stay on track. This little tool is a big motivator for me.

The Butterfly Hop

At one point a young woman just hopped up on the table like a butterfly from one flower to the next. I think this really feeds into a fat person's feelings of inferiority, because I, as a fat person, cannot even attempt this move. I ask you why do previously overweight women do this? I have seen this behavior repeated in other situations. Sunshine, my friend, says they do it because they can. I think it shows a lack of sensitivity to the other members of the group. I hope I never forget how it was for me, so that I can be supportive to others who may need my help and love.

Maybe that butterfly lady started at 140 pounds and reduced to 120 pounds, so in all fairness she really has no idea what it is like to be 200 pounds, just as I have no idea what it is like to be 400 pounds. I didn't feel enriched when I left and I realized that what I was looking for is a "cheerleading" support group that doesn't go out to eat after each meeting. Even if they do, I'll just tell

motion, and that management should do its best to reward a hard working employee.

I'm coming from the "overweight department," which is not really in the company framework that he is talking about, but for me I can see many parallels. Do I believe that I can successfully perform the tasks in front of me? The answer is yes, with lots of hard work. Will this be associated with a positive outcome for me? The answer is yes. Do I believe that what I am working on will have value to me? The answer is yes, in that I will be healthier.

Sharing Thoughts Together

Some of my friends were very kind to share their stories with me. Each one tells me what motivated them to lose weight. My motivation is described in the beginning of this book. It started with the month of insomnia and then the premonition. Vroom's theory is pretty much where I am now, as far as describing to you how I feel. Here are the stories from my friends:

> Dear Kirsten
> "Drive" is a big issue, all-day, everyday. Some days are better than others. The overpowering drive for me is to stave off diabetes, hypertension, and joint problems. To the extent that I am able to control these conditions, I intend to do so. Two years ago, I

was dangerously approaching diagnosis of diabetes and hypertension, and I did experience joint problems when I was heavier. Please understand that I have had a steady creep of weight gain over the past year, despite trying very hard to keep records, avoid processed carbohydrates, live within a fairly narrow daily caloric intake, etc. Now I am exerting every bit of willpower (or "drive") to keep from adding to the problem. To the extent that I can, I avoid potlucks and other situations where I have to look at foods which are particularly tempting to me. Of course, that means a certain loss of social interaction, but I am okay with that. My good friends are "on board" with my new program and we have largely switched to non-food-centered social activities: museum visits, long walks, movies, theater performances, tea or coffee houses, etc.

Hope that helps you. Tammy

Hi Kirsten,

That's fantastic to hear you've lost 19 lbs! That is truly a great accomplishment. It must feel great. I know from experience that kind of weight loss itself becomes a source of motivation for staying on track. I think for me, part of the motivation is knowing that if I veer off track that I'll easily regain the weight I've lost and all the hard work I had done to get here would be lost. Another source of motivation is wanting to be as healthy as I possibly can. I try and remember how good it feels to be healthy, in good shape, physically fit, and in control of my weight.

Now, having said that, I don't always do a great job of staying on track or achieving my weight loss goals. I do struggle with an addiction to carbs, and feel like I could lose 12 or so more pounds. But, I know I've come a long way, and am learning not to beat myself up when I don't eat well, but rather try and seek understanding of what contributes to my own behavior, and work on strategies for improving the chances of success.

I hope this helps answer some of the question... congratulations again on your success so far. Keep up the great work!

Sam

Hi, Kirsten,

For me, my impetus for losing wt was because I didn't want to end up having heart problems like my husband. I didn't want to end up on a respirator. Fear was my reason, and I guess is a big part of trying to keep it off. I guess I feel like I worked hard to get the weight off and learned a lot about how to eat right, so I don't want to lose that progress. Somewhere, too, I don't want to disappoint my doctor and have him tell me that my cholesterol is back up! And I want to be able to fit in my clothes. I have reached the point, where I often prefer

healthy food to junk, but I know that I'm not as good as I used to be. Hope that helps.
love, Maria

I spoke to Maria's husband, who had a heart attack, and he admitted that his biggest reason for losing weight was fear. His heart attack was in 2002, when he weighed 230 pounds. After he recovered, he lost 57 pounds. He did gain a little back.

His story doesn't stand alone. A man at the pool said he was eating junk food and high fat business lunches. At 55 he felt chest pains and went to the hospital, where they told him he needed to lose weight and do some exercise. He hadn't had the heart attack yet, but was on the road in that direction. He started walking and found that as well as exercising in the water, he was actually enjoying himself. He is thankful that he picked up the new habits right away.

Some people are naturally lucky and are born with a perfect metabolism. Lily, my friend, is that way.

Hi Kirsten,
The only time I had to be concerned about my weight was during a couple of my pregnancies. Ordinarily I just seem to burn off the food so that weight gain has never been a major concern. After my last surgery, I put on weight but by the time I discovered that, my

body had begun to shed the pounds -- so basically I've been at the same weight for a zillion years. My shape has changed though. It seems as though older women all develop pot bellies and lose their waistlines. That has happened to me, and while it came as a surprise, I feel that there's nothing I can do about it so I don't really think about it. Validation came when I observed the older women at the pool. Most of us have the pot belly look.
So, you've struck out with me. I have no motivation tips or tidbits to share.
Have a great weekend.
Lily

Hi,
My friends, Dr. Smith and I keep remembering how bad I felt when I was 196 lbs. I want to get back in shape, so I can do the things I used to--ride my bike, dance, garden and feel good about myself. When the weight was on and I couldn't find a Dr. that would listen to me, I became extremely depressed. Then Maria told me about her friend and this new Dr. that helped her friend to lose. I called Dr. Smith's office and not only did she not discount my weight problem and symptoms, but sent me a form for blood work and scheduled me an appointment within the week. This is what I wrote after seeing the Dr. for the first time.

Well, today I found out my test results. Perhaps, if my regular doctor would have performed just one of these tests I wouldn't be in such bad shape. At least things are fixable. In 2003 I weighed 126 lbs. Today at the Dr.'s I weighed 196.9 lbs. (5'5").
Symptoms: Fatigue, sleepiness, weight gain, various aches and pains, depression, inability to think clearly, GI disturbances, hair loss, shortness of breath on exercise, coughing, occasional ringing in ears, headaches, occasional dizziness, irregular heartbeats, and generally a feeling that something is going to kill me if I don't do something.
Just having someone to talk with is inspiring. Dr. Smith still hasn't completely fixed me, but I'm on the road. I know she is doing all she can and together we'll get me back to health. It's the toughest thing I've ever had to do. No one has really researched what happens as we age. It is only recently that people started living this long and combined with modern day hazards, pollutants, etc. there is a lot to learn. Sometimes I feel like her guinea pig, but then I think--at least my granddaughter won't have to feel this way.
I read a lot of books on Thyroid problems, adrenal fatigue, etc and how they effect weight..
Want more--Just write back,
Ursula

Hi Kirsten,
Before losing weight I was an elementary school teacher for 28 years. I had always been a bit "chubby" as a child. I put on the "freshman 15" & never really got rid of it. While dating the man who became my husband, I really started packing it on as our dates mostly consisted of dinners out. I joined Weight Watchers several times, but really got serious when I turned 50. I weighed 203 pounds & only stand 5'1 1/2" tall. My maternal grandmother & mother both had many heart problems. I decided I was heading down the same road & I wanted to do something about it. I joined Weight Watchers in Jan. 2003 when it was offered at my church school. I figured all I had to do was walk down the hall when school was over & attend the meeting. By the fall most people had dropped out, but I continued at other locations. I never actually got to my goal weight, but follow the plan & write a food diary, although not as consistently as before. Since then I've gained back 15 at some point, but am back down to where I was in 2003. It took me 9 months to lose 60 lbs. I basically changed my entire life. When I retired from teaching I wanted to do something else. I started working as a trainer @ Curves in 2005. By then I was up again in part due to abdominal surgery, I lost 20 lbs. in the 2 1/2 years I worked there. Along with the Weight

Watchers program I began to investigate various forms of exercise. I walked at Brookside Gardens. I joined a water aerobics class @ MLK that Maria recommended. I took that class for 3 years & then took the training & became a water aerobics instructor. I now teach 5 days a week, mostly at the Silver Spring Y. I also teach at MLK & I also teach a fitness class to seniors who exercise in their chairs. My main motivation to stay in shape now is because I stand in front of people every day wearing a bathing suit! I also have osteopenia & osteo arthritis in my hips. The best way to keep those under control is do weight bearing exercise for the osteopenia & keep active for the osteoarthritis. Another motivator is the high cost of buying a new wardrobe. I feel good in my clothes now & I have a lot of things I really like. When I was at my heavy weight everything was tight and I had a lot of breathing problems. I got sick a lot, although part of that was being with children all day at school. I used to think it was great if I only got sick once a month. Now I am rarely ever under the weather. Good health has so many benefits that you really appreciate & enjoy when you have them!
I hope that wasn't too much info. Good luck on your journey!
Yoko

What motivates us? For every person it is different. Scolding from doctors doesn't work. They need to focus on the patient's own desire to improve their life. Dr. Smith is helping Ursula. Many doctors don't. I personally think that many of them have given up on us. The person to change our behavior is US. Doctors should give us suggestions, like my last doctor did: "Kirsten, if you were able to lose a considerable amount of weight, you wouldn't have to take so many pills." I am in charge of driving my own car, and not blaming the car for its rusty parts. Ultimately, I need to be accountable to myself; otherwise I will spend my life blaming others.

Fun with My Grandchildren

One of the fun trips that I can remember was going to a berry farm near Santa Cruz with my son and granddaughter. She was excited about posing for photographs, and I have several prints of her standing next to a little red wagon that carried a large box of blackberries that she had "picked." Even though we all did the picking, she was quite proud of them as she told us that she had picked them all.

Capoeira Class

On a couple of Saturdays I went with my family to take my granddaughter to Capoeira Class. This is a Brazilian martial arts type dance class. Watching her and the other children doing this for an hour, I can see that it would be very exhausting. Another activity in which my little grandson was too young to participate was the pre-school Halloween parade. My little granddaughter was at the head of the line holding the teacher's hand. She was dressed as the most beautiful witch I have ever seen. For Halloween, my little grandson did have a Dalmatian suit that he wore that night. The world seems to have a special sparkle to it when you have grandchildren.

On the celebrity side of the news, Tiger Woods was wrapped up in his own scandal, one that he truly made himself. He had a beautiful wife but also had 15 mistresses at different locations, who stepped forward, one after the other, to tell their stories on the television news. The famous golfer admitted he had let his family down, and then one month later resumed his golf tournaments.

The rest of the world wasn't doing that great, either. Far more oil spilled into the Gulf of Mexico than they ever anticipated. In just a month, starting in April 2010, 30 million gallons had poured into the Gulf. This disaster went on for months. President Obama told us he was "dealing" with the British Petroleum officials. The beaches were becoming dirty on the Louisiana coast. Tourism was drying up. Katrina had hit them, and now it was the Gulf Oil Spill's turn. How much more could these poor people take?

Earthquake and Tsunami

Another disaster struck when an 8.9 earthquake hit Japan on March 11, 2011. It was 900 times more powerful than the Loma Prieta earthquake of l989 that I experienced.

The California earthquake happened on October 17, 1989 and was referred to as the "World Series Earthquake." It was centered along the San Andreas Fault in the San Francisco Bay Area. On the Richter scale it was 6.9 or, as we were later told, it was a 7.1 earthquake. We definitely felt it. Our cat gave me a dirty look, as if to say, "Why did you do that?"

Japan's earthquake was much, much worse. I saw a video on television where a chandelier shook violently, not just a gentle sway as I had seen in 1989. After that terrible event in Japan, there was a tsunami that followed. It hit Japan, Hawaii and the West Coast of the United States. Aerial photos showed muddy waters surging through Japan, taking the people, the houses and the cars in one giant grab. It was so sad to see this devastation.

Then, as if all that wasn't bad enough, they had to fear radiation leaks from the Fukushima Nuclear Power Plant (April 27, 2011). I observed the resilience of a Japanese man when I heard him say, "We can't look backward, we need to look forward." That shows courage and unbelievable strength.

A story of great national pride comes to mind during the year after we returned from Georgia. This was when the Chilean miners were rescued from one of their mines on October 13, 2010. I found that I wanted to watch the stories over and over, to see the men greeted by cheers and embraces from their families. Thirty-three miners were rescued, one at a time, into the daylight. The whole world was cheering for them, not just their country, and not just America.

When the November/December holidays came around, we had our special "Thanksmas" celebration. This was invented because my son and his wife were going to spend Christmas with her parents in Brazil, and wouldn't return home until January 6, 2011. We had Christmas toys that we wanted to give to our grandchildren, but not in January. Some of the gifts they received were pillow pets, a robot movie, a gumball machine, a shopping cart and a fire truck. They played with their toys until it was time for them to go home and go to sleep.

I spent Christmas Eve visiting my daughter and son-in-law. We went to a steak restaurant in San Francisco, and to Macy's in Union Square to see the Christmas lights. The day after Christmas I visited my friend Sunshine, her husband, her sons, her daughter-in-law and her little grandson. Christmas is more than the presents and the tree; it is the wonderful feeling that we feel in our hearts that gives us joy.

Discussing Weight Issues with Edgar

My friend, Edgar, called me yesterday to tell me about a play called "Forty Pounds in Twelve Weeks: A Love Story." It is a one-woman comedy show, being held at the Marsh in San Francisco. The woman comedian tells of her battle with her overbearing father, a gymnastics coach, who threatened her with not paying for her college education if she didn't lose 40 pounds over the summer. She has done the American weight gain and weight loss yo-yo, like many of us have. The show focuses on her weight issues, not her thin self. The reviewer didn't really care much for the play, saying it was more of an exercise of "pity" than a comedy. (SF Weekly.com)

This subject ties into a television show about overweight people called "The Biggest Loser." Edgar and I have been discussing this show. NBC is in its fourth season showing this program.

When I asked some friends what they thought of this television program, I got several different answers. One lady said, "Oh, they are so brave." Another lady said, "I worry about them; they exercise so hard; I guess they have doctors there; what if a contestant were to collapse?" Still another lady said, "I sure hope someone doesn't drop dead on the show from eating only a 1,000 calories and exercising four to five hours a day."

I'm not a big game show or survival show type person, but as this show fits in with my struggle with weight, I decided to watch it a few times. Sixteen people are gathered at the weight loss ranch in Malibu, where trainers work with them. At the end of the show, the grand winner, (the biggest loser), gets $250,000 for the first prize. Whoever has the least amount of weight loss gets voted off each week. The men are often between 300 and 400 pounds and the women are between 200 and 300 pounds when they begin the program.

A two pound weight loss per week, which would be a "healthy" weight loss, would get a person eliminated from the show. The show focuses in on two areas. One is exercise, and the other is diet. What I don't like about the show is the extremely large weight loss rates, five to seven pounds a week, which is not realistic for the average person at home. This might discourage the viewer when he can't lose weight as rapidly as the people on the television show. They might give up and think that the only way for them to achieve their goals is to get on the show.

The reality is that weight loss is a "slow and steady" race that requires patience and hard work.

Does the show tell Mr. and Ms. America that in order to get healthy they must do 500 squats, 50 laps, and 10 mile runs as often as possible to stay fit? The message I read is that if we don't work our bodies to the breaking point, we will never become successful in our weight loss.

My friend Edgar says that we must remember, "It's a game show, like Wheel of Fortune, or Jeopardy." Some of the contestants win; some of them lose. Actually, the real prize is not the money; it is the pounds that you lose. Edgar says the real object of the show is to get people to watch and purchase the products advertised in the commercials, like low calorie microwave meals or high fiber cereal.

The white team, the blue team, the red team, and the black team compete against each other. I feel the show sometimes isn't completely honest. As an example, there was an Easter egg hunt, and there was one "golden egg," which the contestants were told was the prize worth "more than anything" that each of them would want. Many of the players thought it was money. It turned out that the "golden egg" prize was the privilege "to vote someone off the show." I would have felt tricked. That is not the prize I would have wanted the most.

Edgar says the show is "insightful," because they talk about diet, exercise and mental attitude. To keep the game going, he says it is impossible to predict who is going to win at the end. Many of the contestants are happy going home with their weight loss, but Edgar thinks that some of the really competitive people in the show are out to win the prize money.

He told me that he saw in the beginning where the doctors told a 26 year old contestant that he might be 26 years old, but that his body was really that of a 54 year old. Edgar said the show is a frank discussion about people's weight issues, and not just a critical finger pointing at them. He said he thought you could learn from the show, but that it is not always reality.

Twice I saw on the show where the contestants had to strap the weight that they lost back on themselves, and exercise while wearing the weight. It is hard to carry that extra weight around once you have given it up. This is an example to show the contestants that they may wish to never gain that weight back. I was thinking about that. What would it be like if I strapped five five-pound bags of sugar on my back and went around doing my daily chores carrying that extra weight? I know it would be hard.

Another lady I talked to about the program told me she lost 50 pounds twice, once as a teenager, and the second time after the birth of her third and last child. She said she was concerned about the way the contestants have such hard workouts, and she thinks they will have joint problems later in life because of these workouts. I can get joint problems with mild workouts, so I understand what she is saying.

As I said at the beginning, "Those people are very brave."

The Brave Revolutionary American

Bravery is not something for the weak of heart. The news coming out of North Africa shows an American revolutionary spirit. I saw an article in Newsweek, March 7, 2011, by Niall Ferguson asking, "So why are Americans cheering on the Arab revolutionary wave?"

The author is a learned man, but in my opinion, he doesn't totally feel the pulse of what made America great. We fought off an oppressive ruler, the King of England, who was out to take all he could from a continent an ocean away. We fought to establish our own political order, and the process didn't come overnight. There were years of oppression and "taxation without representation," which came prior to our revolution. We knew that fighting would be needed to achieve our goals.

Sure, we had some very intelligent leaders, but who is to say that some learned men won't step up in Africa. From my travels, I learned the world is different every place you go, but the desire for freedom is much the same. I do not agree with the author when he says that Americans should just stick to loving their own revolution.

As I watched television I was supporting the people of Egypt in their quest for democracy. By changing the channels, I found I could watch Al Jazeera English on DirecTV. Some Americans think this is the voice of terrorists, but they are doing an excellent job of covering the news of North Africa.

Each day on the news I saw the people of Egypt protesting against their leader, Hosni Mubarak. Al Jazeera said the average person in Egypt has very low wages. They were fighting for a better life. U.S. officials are worried about who will follow after Mubarak. But to do nothing, and sit in fear in a house ruled by a tyrant, is not an acceptable way to live.

If you never lift a foot you will never go anywhere. To make any kind of progress, a person needs to take decisive action to do something.

Actually, I waited until it was almost too late to embark on my quest of losing weight. I already have diabetes, and some joint problems in my knees, but I am taking action and moving forward.

There Are Also Mountains in Libya

Egypt didn't have the brutal bloodshed that I see happening now in Libya. The big difference is that Hosni Mubarak is not Colonel Muammar el-Qaddafi. Colonel Qaddafi will kill all his opponents, not stopping until he is left ruling only the sand of his country.

Four New York Times journalists were freed from Libya. I read the account of their ordeal. One of them reported he heard his captors yell, "Shoot them." Another captor said, "No, they're American, we can't shoot them." The woman of the group said that every man she came in contact with grabbed her breasts. One soldier threatened one of the journalists, and told him he was going to be decapitated.

Luckily, they are free now, but another 13 journalists are missing or are in custody. Many of the rebels have been shot. What worked in Egypt doesn't appear to be working in Libya. Will Libya get its democracy and a new leader?

Tip # 18
"In Every Walk with Nature One Receives More Than He Seeks."
–John Muir

A week of daily rain has finally stopped and the sun has emerged. As I took my walk I saw a 200 foot strip of purple ice plant in full bloom. After I had walked the distance, I turned around to feast my eyes on it once more. I watched as another "exercise" walker, with his earphones on, didn't glance at the ice plant at all. He was just advancing as fast as he could. He didn't even look, not even once, at nature's beauty. There is more to life than just exercising.

On my walks I keep meeting new neighbors, now that it is spring. The man next door has a model airplane that he works on. He told me I could take my grandson to a local high school on Sundays to see people flying their planes. I know a little two-year old that would love that.

My Spirits Are Getting Inflated

Meeting my mailman at his truck several doors down, I was surprised when he said, "Hello, Mrs. Crabill." I asked him if he had lost any weight after starting the job and he said, "I started at

205 pounds, and after 30 days I was approaching 155 pounds." He said it was a new route for him, plus a new job, which was stressful. He told me he walked from nine in the morning until four in the afternoon. Once he became familiar with the route his weight jumped to 170 pounds, where it has stayed. He mentioned he is a diabetic who also has a thyroid problem, for which his doctor gives him medication.

When I told him that I have to be very careful what I eat he said, "Oh no, I just eat whatever I want, but not lots of cakes." It is the "whatever I want" part that intrigued me. I had eaten "whatever I want" when I wasn't dieting for 60 years and ballooned to 220 pounds. Now my balloon is getting deflated, and my spirits are getting inflated.

Workers Suffering Weight Stigma

Talking about my mailman made me think of all the workers in America. David and I are retired now, but we used to be among them. I have gone through hard times in a job when I was discriminated against because I was pregnant, but I've never encountered weight discrimination as an issue. Susie Q told me she had worked at a fabric store. She did get hired, but found out later she was the last one considered when it came to scheduling days off. The thinner employees always got asked first when the manager was making the schedule. Essentially, she got what was left. She wanted to keep her job, so she just accepted it.

She was a nice person, and very knowledgeable about fabrics, but she was noticeably overweight. For this, she wore her scarlet letter. As she stood at the cutting counter she could hear the other female employees making crude remarks about her. She had good suggestions, such as eliminating the tractor print fabrics, as the store was in a suburban area, but the manager never listened to her input.

"Weight stigma" is where the overweight person feels he has received unfair treatment. He feels others are poking fun at him because of his size. I have read that often thin people think fat people are unmotivated, lazy and stupid. This is totally absurd. The issue is extra layers of fat, not a shortage of brain cells.

This stigma happens not only at the workplace, but also on college campuses, at healthcare facilities, and I have unfortunately seen it at gyms. During exercise class the new girl was not referred to by her name, but behind her back she was called, "the fat girl." Maybe they didn't know her name during her first month of visits, but why did this name calling continue after that? I have seen other new thin girls come into the class, but the others quickly addressed her by name.

The fat stigma permeates all people in our society. We are now more "weight conscious," but we are also more "weight critical." Unfortunately, there are no laws against this bias, and it continues to thrive. It can take the form of verbal teasing and derogatory remarks.

The fatter a person is, the more they are the target of "fat jokes." When I was handing out my weight survey in the locker room, the ladies treated me like an equal, even though at that point I was just less than 200 pounds.

I will always remember the new "fat girl" that joined the class. I befriended her right away, because I didn't want her to feel the pain of "fat stigma." I always enjoyed her company and never labeled her. To me it was important that she felt like she had a friend. Susie Q left the gym, but if I ever see her again, I plan to continue our relationship, since "size has nothing to do with friendship."

Workers Suffering Weight Discrimination

More serious than weight stigma is weight discrimination. This is where a person gets fired from a job because that person is labeled as "too overweight." Behind closed doors the words said are: that person is "too fat." This is real discrimination, no different than age discrimination or sex discrimination.

Why is it okay to have negative attitudes toward overweight people? Unfortunately, there are not many laws to protect overweight people. The Rehabilitation Act of 1973 and the Americans with Disabilities Act of 1990 are two places where victims can turn for help with weight discrimination.

The problem is that these laws focus on "morbidly obese" people, so if you are just overweight, you have no "legal" ground to stand on. Not many cases have a successful outcome when the overweight person takes his or her "discrimination case" to court.

The following are laws and local ordinances concerning discrimination:

The Rehabilitation Act of 1973 prohibits discrimination against an otherwise qualified individual with handicaps, solely on the basis of that handicap, in any program which receives federal assistance.

The Americans with Disabilities Act of 1990 extends the protection against discrimination on the basis of disability to the private sector.

The State of Michigan bans discrimination in employment based on race, color, religion, national origin, age, sex, height, weight, or marital status.

Santa Cruz, California (July 1992) defines unlawful discrimination as "differential treatment as a result of that person's race, color, creed, religion, national origin, ancestry, disability, marital status, sex gender, sexual orientation, height, weight, or physical characteristic."

District of Columbia (Human Rights Law) outlaws discrimination, also listing "personal appearance, and physical handicap."

San Francisco, California (June 2000) outlaws discrimination against people based on their weight. The Council on Size and Weight Discrimination www.cswd.org

I saw a list of 31 court cases from the "Aele Law Library of Case Summaries." About 10 of them were awarded in the overweight person's favor. Discrimination is really hard to prove, and even more so to have a "law" that will protect you.

When I talked to friends at the gym, one said that she didn't know any cases of weight discrimination during her years working as a professional. The other friend said that once she applied for a job as a church secretary, she listed on her application that her "negative qualities" were that she liked to "eat under stress." She said she got the job anyway, although I have to wonder whether it was because she was so well qualified, since she had been a school teacher prior to her retirement.

Many people don't win their lawsuits. Companies are very clever and have clauses in their work contracts. These include certain "appearance standards" that must be met. They can also say that the worker "did not meet the minimum physical requirements." They can be very selective and when there are several applicants equally qualified to stock shelves at the hardware store, they would most likely pick the tallest one, as he may not need to get a ladder as often.

My friend Edgar said that policemen and firemen often are hired in their 20s or 30s, when they are slim. These same men could now be in their 40s and 50s and showing some middle age weight gain.

To win in court against a company that has more resources than just one person is hard. The following is a court case in 1991 that took place in New Jersey.

Gimello v. Agency Rent-A-Car Systems Inc.
250 NJ Super

[250 NJSuper Page 340]

...the complainant, Joseph Gimello, claimed he was a victim of discriminatory discharge from employment. He claimed he was fired because of his obesity, a condition unrelated to his ability to do his job.

[250 NJSuper Page 341]

His employer claimed he was terminated "because of inadequate job performance." The Director of the Division of Civil Rights, confirming the findings of the administrative law judge, concluded that the employer's reason for termination was pretextual, not bona fide, and that Gimello really was fired because of his actual or perceived obesity and not for any legitimate business reason.

[250 NJSuper Page 343]

written in the margin. On the memo showing the office's 100 percent sales quota "average through February 13, 1979" DPC sales, Thatcher wrote: "Joe: OUTSTANDING ... WHAT ELSE CAN I SAY. THANKS. JIM T." In March 1979 Thatcher wrote: JOE: THIS IS A COMPANY ALL TIME RECORD – INCREDIBLE JOB. JIM

[250 NJSuper Page 345]

...Memo dated December 8, 1981, described Gimello as a "good" office manager, but conditioned a recommendation for promotion on Gimello's taking a "course in employee/public relations."...Memo dated May 1, 1982, ...Mogar noted that Gimello should soften his telephone skills with customers...

[250 NJSuper Page 345]

...Mogar told Brindisi that he felt Gimello was "promotable to a district manager's spot." Mogar testified that Brindisi said, "I don't feel Joe is promotable because of his size and weight." Mogar stated that Brindisi thought that Gimello would not be able to travel from office to office to perform a district manager's functions. Mogar stated that at first he laughed because he thought Brindisi was joking but he later realized that Brindisi was serious.

[250 NJSuper Page 346]

Gimello was "surprised" but "handled it kind of lightly" because he felt his "track record would stand for itself."

As Gimello reflected on Brindisi's comment, he decided to try to lose weight. He consulted Dr. Samuel Goldman, a specialist of 30 years in the field of weight loss on February 7, 1983...Gimello lost 52 pounds by May 1983.

Goldman testified at the hearing both as a treating physician and as an expert in the field of treating obesity....Goldman stated that while overeating, heredity and metabolism were factors that might cause obesity, pinpointing the exact cause of any patient's obesity is difficult....In Goldman's opinion, Gimello's weight did not impede his ability to perform his job. He said: "Mr. Gimello has been obese the majority of his life, and I doubt very much that it has been a detriment to his work in any way. It has no bearing on his ability to perform his duties."

[250 NJSuper Page 347]

...Mogar testified that when Gimello returned to the front of the office to assist customers, Garrenton told him that Gimello was the cause of the problem "because of his size and appearance." Garrenton pointed to Gimello through a window between the offices and said, "that's your problem over there, that fat slob."...

[250 NJSuper Page 348]

...When Gimello would not resign, [after being asked] Mogar fired him on June 9, 1983 at Brindisi's direction....He was fired for "Not providing the service to our customers."....Four days later, Agency fired Gimello's wife, Terri, from her part-time job in the Cherry Hill office.

[250 NJSuper Page 351]

After he was fired on June 9, 1983, Gimello found another job about 1 ½ years later, in October 1984.... The State Division of Unemployment sent Gimello a "notice of determination" which read:

"You were terminated June 9, 1983 because management felt you were not promotable. There had been no complaints about your work. You worked to the best of your ability."...

Gimello testified that he actively sought another job but had difficulty because prospective employers thought that he must have done something wrong to get fired.... Gimello stopped seeing Dr. Goldman because he could not afford to pay him. As a result, he claimed he regained the weight lost. Both Gimello and his wife testified to the financial difficulties the family experienced following his termination.

[250 NJSuper Page 355]

...We conclude that the record adequately supports the factual findings of the legal conclusion that Gimello was a victim of discrimination because of his obesity.

I don't know the actual number of cases related to weight stigma or weight discrimination, as many never make it to court. Also, I don't know how many men over 50, who have been looking for work, were not offered positions because of their age. Many cases of discrimination go unreported.

Tip # 19
"Injustice Anywhere Is a Threat
To Justice Everywhere."
–Dr. Martin Luther King, Jr.

Thirty Pound Loss

I'll just look at the number on the scale, and not think about my new 46.2 percent body fat number. When the pencil remarked that I had lost 30 pounds, I could see instant amazement and respect that came in my direction. I'm the same person as before, only now I get more recognition than I did in the beginning. Fat people don't get any recognition and often very little respect. See what happens when you lose 30 pounds.

One lady who hardly spoke to me before said, "Wow! You lost 30 pounds!" Another lady who I said "Hi" to in the locker room, a week after I started the class, barely responded to me. When I asked her, "Do you know who I am?" She said, "Yes," and that she was in a hurry. Why didn't she just say "Hi" to me the first time? We talked a little after my 30 pound weight loss was announced. Am I more exciting to know, now that I have lost 30 pounds?

Another lady, who I don't know, and who I didn't even see as I was looking down in my purse to get my car keys, said within earshot of me, "Let's see if she can keep it off." I didn't want to look up to see who said such a mean remark. I do have a quote for her.

"The Higher We Soar the Smaller We Appear To Those Who Cannot Fly." –Friedrich Nietzsche

There are 14 people who came for the follow-up weight loss class. They discussed that if you can hold your weight for three years you will most likely maintain it. At the scale it wasn't so good for me today. I had lost four pounds and the same teacher who had announced last week that I had lost 30 pounds told me I had lost too much weight. My weight loss should have been no more than three pounds.

One lady in the group said, "Oh, you shouldn't work so hard on trying to lose weight." Another lady said, "The teacher is just concerned about your health and losing weight too fast." Maybe next week I won't lose so much and the teacher will be pleased.

Today I went to the gym where I do water exercises, and spoke to a good friend about my weight loss. She hugged me. Then she said, looking straight at me, "I know how very hard it is," and then gave me another hug. How sad it is that I have to go to another place to get support.

We each received a food to take home and prepare. Unfortunately, I burned the pot with my lentil mixture. Cooking does not hold the fascination for me that it once did.

Halfway through the class the teachers traded places, each one teaching in the room where she hadn't been before. More concepts were introduced. Some of the ladies had been showing their upper arms to the teacher and asked what they could do to lose fat in this area. The teacher said we cannot "spot" reduce, thus we may still have "wings" under our arms. Where we lose weight is genetically determined.

The other students then spoke of their goals. Once everyone had spoken, the teacher mentioned that exercise makes a person feel better. Months ago, one student said, "The best exercise is the one that works for you."

Everyone left quickly, but I waited and went into the other class to find a lady who was at my original class. She had been very friendly to me before, and her absence made me sad.

A smile came to my face when I was driving home as I followed a car that had a license plate holder that said:

**"Hand Over The Chocolate
AND NOBODY GETS HURT!"**

I missed the next class and was very thankful when Harriet e-mailed notes to me. Harriet had always been very quiet toward me, so I was really surprised when I opened her e-mail. Maybe I had been too critical about the lack of support that I was feeling. That was kindness on her part, and I personally thanked her the next time I saw her.

The Most Powerful Weight Loss Tool

I left the house to take my walk. The sky was dark but I thought I could try my luck. Raindrops stopped me as soon as I began my walk. This turned out to be my opportunity to fix myself some Earl Grey tea. Tea tastes especially good when it is raining.

Reaching up in the cupboard toward my assortment of mugs, I pulled out a mug that honored its user by saying, "The Only Person Who Really Knows What's Going On." I chuckled, as it is so true. Only my mind and I know what I am doing. The mind is the most powerful weight loss tool we have.

Tip # 20
"A Mind Is Like A Parachute. It Doesn't Work If It Is Not Open."
–Frank Zappa

Answers.com says the mind has 70,000 thoughts on an average day. There are 86,400 seconds in a 24 hour day. That means we have a different thought every 1.2 seconds.

I decided to do my own little test to demonstrate this statement to be correct. I was going to do it all day, only I found it difficult to record all of my thoughts. Just thinking about me thinking about it was exhausting.

Starting at 10:00 a.m. these were my thoughts:

- Do this experiment.
- Go to the kitchen – did the math – thinking how nice it would be to lose three pounds this week.
- Take a shower.
- How nice the hot water feels on my shoulders.
- How green the bottle of shampoo is.
- Wipe off the water bubbles on my arm.

- Put my husband's partially eaten apple pie back in its wrapper.
- The rain is tapping on my kitchen window.
- Need to get dressed.
- Want one drink of diet coke.
- Plan to go to the library at 11:00 a.m.
- Just want a second sip of diet coke.

Took a break to rest with my husband (bleep, bleep, bleep - you can't read this part).

- Getting up I wonder should I wear white or black socks.
- Oh, I need to take my pills before I forget.
- Need to put a little conditioner on my hair, it sure looks dry.
- Want to watch more of "Cleopatra," the movie with Elizabeth Taylor, as she died yesterday. She is so beautiful. I'm working on being the best I can be, but I'll never be Elizabeth Taylor.
- Want to study information to include in my book.
- Am fixing my hair. I need a quick clean-up of my bathrooms.
- Never want to wear any second-hand clothes from a lady who sells them as her

"fat" clothes. Have done this twice in my life.

- Am going to the kitchen to eat one prune, my new candy.
- Need to put coins in plastic Easter eggs for my grandchildren. Parents don't want jellybeans.
- Am wondering, as I am filling the eggs, are the children going to covet money now and not candy?
- New printer works like a high-speed bullet train.
- Old printer works like a horse.
- Now I'm thinking my thoughts are jumping all over the place.
- (I'm reading a magazine.) Thinking about a man who organized rag pickers in India to help them turn garbage into fuel. (Saw this photo with the above caption.) Wow. Some people are so giving of themselves.
- Am feeling selfish just trying to work on improving myself.
- Maybe the next step is helping the poor in India. No, that's not really me.
- (Husband is driving me to the library.) I'm watching the splash coming up from the tires of the cars.

- Am tired. Have looked through probably 50 books at the library book sale. Many books seem to be on Iraq and Afghanistan.
- Found the self-help section. Am looking through the brain books.
- I'm enjoying the turkey/avocado sandwich that I'm eating for lunch.
- Am listening to the Adventures of a Man in Baja, Mexico on the car radio.
- Can't get out of the car, even though we are home, until the story is over.
- Thinking about how hard it is to write down all my thoughts. It is 1:00 p.m. and I've started all this thinking at 10:00 a.m. I'm exhausted with thinking about all my thinking. I haven't even recorded all my thoughts. This exercise is ending soon. I'm tired.

Here is a thought I forgot to write while at the library. I saw a book on "How to Marry the Perfect Man," but I didn't buy it. I already have the perfect man. I told my husband and he said, "Did you see the book on 'What to Do with Your Lazy Husband?'" We both laughed. My thought now is to get back to writing the book.

You should do this half-day exercise just once. It is so exhausting. You might laugh about all the things you think about. I didn't include some of the ridiculous details. Once I was looking at the bedroom door-frame and thought how nicely it was squared off. My thoughts just seem to jump all over the place.

I just did a fast clean-up of the bath-rooms, so I won't be thinking about having to do that chore all afternoon. I wanted to stop those bathroom thoughts from nagging me.

Sweep Away the Negative Thoughts

Fear and panic can give us energy. Some of the people I know, myself included, are moved to lose weight because of fear of an unhealthy future. No one wants heart prob-lems or knee problems. Sometimes fear can cripple you into uncertainty.

When I was five years old as I was walking down the street with my father, a large Ger-man shepherd ran out from a neighbor's yard and jumped on me. The owner apolo-gized to my father, but the damage had been done. The rest of that long, hot summer we kept some bedroom windows closed. Even though we lived on the second floor, I was positive that dog could fly up and enter our home through the windows of our apartment. Fear overtook my rational brain. When you are an adult you have lived longer and are better able to use your knowledge to help you and not imprison you.

It is best not to think that you are the victim, although many people do this. When walls come crashing down on you, I can understand how you feel. I just heard that Japan has had the second earthquake after the first 9.1 quake which was followed by the tsunami. I can easily see how these people would feel like they are victims. I see it as being so unfair. Haven't they had enough? I don't understand. I wish the survivors courage to help them pull through.

To make progress in our life we need to clean house. We need to take the broom and sweep the negative thoughts out the door. We need to pack up, donate, or throw away the extra mental baggage that is sitting in the closets of our minds collecting dust and haunting us. There is no room in the closet to put the positive thoughts if the negative ones are occupying too much space.

The main tool you need when you go on any new meal plan is to use your mind. Before I ever signed up for the weight loss class, my mind had been made up: This time it was for real, for keeps, not just to fit in a pretty dress for my daughter's wedding, or to shed a few pounds before getting pregnant. All of those steps were just the "before" steps, and once the goal was reached there was no incentive to stay on track. Why my total well-being wasn't enough, I don't know, but all the other times I just took the "before" steps.

The Before and After Photo

There are weight loss tips written everywhere, in magazines, newspapers and on the web. These are the "before" and "after," and the "all the time" guidelines. Be realistic and patient. Create a routine and stop making excuses. Here are a few of my rules. Use your mind to keep you from drifting. Educate yourself using your mind to make better choices. Commit to your plan: "This one is forever."

When you feel weak, drill positive thoughts into your mind over and over like a skipping record: I CAN DO IT. Your mind has the power. When all the electricity in the world fails, your mind energizes you toward success. You know there will be a lot of distractions. Use *your mind to click the switch in the correct direction. After the lectures, the books and the teachers, when you go home and are all alone, it's your mind that can be your friend and help you make the right decision. That's what friends are for.*

I am closing this section with a little verse, quoting from the Goethe Society of North America. [Mutti used to tell me that I was related to Goethe, through my maternal line, although I have no way to prove it.] This verse was translated by John Anster from Goethe's Faust, written in 1835. It shows how a doubting mind can transform into a positive one.

"Then indecision brings its own delays,
And days are lost lamenting over lost days.
Are you in earnest? Seize this very minute;
What you can do, or dream you can do, begin it;
Boldness has genius, power and magic in it."

This morning I went shopping, as some of my clothes are getting too large for me. I bought two blouses that have a little tighter fit than I would like, thus I can't overeat and gain the weight back. That statement is just a cover up, because your mind has to be in the right place even if you don't buy a new blouse.

One Hundred Twenty Percent

We came home and mowed the lawn. By then I was really tired. I grabbed a half-eaten bag of carrot chips; those special ones that are ready to eat. As I sat there I closed my eyes and listened to the crunch, crunch, crunch of the carrots, and felt good that I was eating. I finished off the second half of the 16 ounce bag. When there were no more carrots to put in my mouth, I flipped the plastic bag over and started to read it. It said zero, zero, zero percent on the fats. Sodium was three percent, and then I got down farther on the list to Vitamin A and it said 120 percent. Wow! One hundred twenty percent of whatever made me feel so good. When I am tired, a 120 percent boost spurs me on to a really happy afternoon.

"No Turning Back"
–General Ulysses S. Grant

Today is April 12, 2011, the 150 year anniversary of the start of the American Civil War. Many new books have come out. When I was watching C-Span Book TV, I saw a clip as I was walking through the living room. James Perry, the author of *A Bohemian Brigade,* was talking about Civil War correspondents. He said that General Grant told a reporter, "This time there will be no turning back," and to give that message to Lincoln. That is how it has to be with weight loss.

James Madison, who was born on March 16, 1751, was our smallest President, weighing only 100 pounds and standing five feet four inches tall. The writer Washington Irving once described him as "but a withered little Apple-John."

Our largest President, William Taft, born September 15, 1857, was nicknamed "Big Bill." He stood six feet two inches and weighed 350 pounds. Once he got stuck in the White House bathtub, and had a new one installed that was large enough to hold four men. He died when he was 73 years old, due to arteriosclerotic heart disease, high blood pressure and inflammation of the bladder.

Michelle Obama, President Obama's wife, is promoting healthy eating among our children. Her family came from the village of Rex, Georgia, close to where we lived. A New York Times article said there was a young slave girl who was impregnated by a white man, and these two people are the great-great-great grandparents of Michelle Obama. When I think of the people who have risen up in the world, and when I see their humble roots, I have nothing but respect for their hard work.

Michelle Obama's aim is to help American families eat more nutritious food. In her program she is first focusing on the children. The new standards would not remove a popular food like pizza from the school menu, but an effort will be made to make pizza healthier by using whole wheat crust and low-fat mozzarella cheese. Vending machines would have water and healthier juices instead of high calorie sodas. She wants to empower the families and their communities to make better food choices. Her goal is to improve school lunches, distribute nutritional education to families, and get the school children to move more.

Her ideas are to help the children develop good habits. They can pass these ideas on to their children and this terrible obesity crisis that we are in (which started about 1970 and has been going on for 40 years) could cease to become a problem. Effective advertising about the perils of smoking drastically reduced the number of smokers. Children grow up now knowing smoking is bad for their health, which is a far cry from the 1940s sexy smoking movie stars. I applaud Mrs. Obama.

I heard about Kym St. Clair, who owns the Curves franchise at Foxworthy and Union Avenues in San Jose. She says she has struggled with weight all her life, and wanted to do something to help herself and others. She adopts the ladies that come to her club who later become her faithful exercise family.

Charity is an important part of her life, and she has her clients get involved with her to help others. She once put a large suitcase in the middle of the exercise floor, where people could bring in children's shoes that they shipped to Haiti. They held a baby shower for the single mothers at San Jose's Heritage House. They all got together and sent cookies and snack food to our soldiers overseas. It doesn't end there. She is a lady who just keeps on giving as she is keeping herself and her clients fit.

Contemporary American Life: Fast Food

Currently fast foods are "Evil" and are blamed for the obesity crisis. Like many Americans, I have feasted on hamburgers layered with cheese and bacon, and ordered French fries. For only 20 cents more I could maximize my soda. Part of that behavior has gotten me in this mess.

But in defense of the fast food industry, some of them have now introduced low calorie choices. At Taco Bell I have eaten the Fresco Chicken Soft Taco, 150 calories; at Subway I have eaten the Six Inch Turkey Breast Sandwich, 280 calories; and at Wendy's I have eaten the half chicken salad, 340 calories. Fast food places are making an effort to take a more nutritional stance by offering some low calorie options. I read that only 25 percent of Americans even look or consider the low calorie options, but I do. And, by the way, I've lost 30 pounds by eating lunches at the places I mentioned.

There are many articles in the news on how to turn the obesity problem around. I was shocked to hear that the Arizona Governor wants to "revamp the Medicaid Program" by making some drastic changes. Governor Jan Brewer is proposing to place fees on adults who lead unhealthy lives. This is to cover "Childless adults who are obese or suffer from a chronic condition and who fail to work with their doctor to meet specific goals. They would be charged $50 annually. The $50 annual fee would also apply to all childless adult smokers."

The point is that if you are going to cost the state money, you should be responsible and take action, so that you won't cost the state as much money. People on Medicaid do not have lots of money. It is much cheaper to feed yourself on the fast food special, no matter how many calories it has, than to go to the market and buy one basket of cherry tomatoes for $3.99. What about vouchers they can use to help them buy the healthy food? Fifty dollars for them is a lot, and for the government it is very little, compared to the long term medical costs associated with obesity. No one wins here, not the poor person, not the government.

Most poor people have television sets. Maybe they even watch "The Biggest Loser." I find it very motivational. I'll never be the biggest loser like on the show, but I am working hard just like they are.

Rulan, the Olympic Gold Medal Champion wrestler who was on the show, lost 144 pounds. Here is someone Americans can look up to. He celebrated his victory for too long by eating too many pizzas. He is brave to be on the program.

Give the poor people extra discount vouchers with their food stamps so that they will be drawn to eat more healthy fruits and vegetables. Local gyms should offer, by lottery, free memberships that will be considered a tax write-off by the government. Do these things instead of a $50 fine.

For every person out there that is trying to lose weight I want to share the following:

"Every job is a portrait of the person who does it. Autograph your work with excellence."
–Author Unknown

My life and my struggles, my thoughts and my food, and my enlightenment from the course and study, are all woven into the braid of this book. I am working toward ex-

cellence. I know losing weight is hard. I also know that keeping it off will be the same challenge.

I spoke to my good friend, Henry, whom I haven't seen for a long time. He is really tall, six feet six inches, and he is very heavy at 500 pounds. He gave me permission to print our telephone interview.

The Wonderful World of the Thin

I asked him if he could wake up tomorrow and be thin would he want this to happen. Then I asked him to explain why. He answered, "I wish I could wake up to be the appropriate weight for my height. That would be wonderful. As difficult as it is to lose weight, it is even harder to keep it off. Now I'm in the worst of all possible worlds, almost totally incapacitated. There is no effective way that I can exercise."

When I mentioned to him about his extraordinary height, he said all the people on his father's side were tall, and many of the people on his mother's side were farmers from the Midwest. He told me that it's really hard for him to buy clothes that fit, "As, if you are male, you are either supposed to be tall and skinny, or short and fat."

"I have a disability in that I have nerve damage on the right side of my body, which makes it difficult for me to walk. The less I walk, the more my muscles lose their strength, and this makes it again more difficult to walk.

"It is terribly difficult for me to get into automobiles, which makes me more housebound. The doctors are after me all the time to lose weight. I get annoyed that no matter what is wrong with me the doctor says it is because of my weight."

Then I talked to him about gastric bypass surgery. He said, "I noticed that Al Roker did that after he got married, so I think Al's wife started it all." On gastric bypass he said, "It's a big lifestyle change. You have to think about why are you eating so much, and if the answer is simply because you are hungry, then the gastric bypass will work, because your stomach is much smaller and you will feel full faster. If you eat for other reasons, not just hunger, it will not work.

"Before I would consider doing this type of surgery I will have to think, would I be able to make it work in the long run? One of the things I have been wondering about is a fast, like a week-long fast, to shrink my stomach to get the process going for weight loss. That would be where I eat nothing, but drink liquids and vitamins, and it would have to be supervised by an M.D.

"I believe heavy men face less discrimination than women, but I have personally faced discrimination from upper management because of my size. I have seen less qualified people get the position simply because of their thinner front desk appearance."

SEVERELY OVERWEIGHT FEEL WORST TREATMENT

Rates of perceived weight/height discrimination among U.S. adults ages 25-74:

Percentage:

Weight status	Men	Women
Normal weight	2.2	2.2
Overweight	3.5	8.6
Moderately obese	6.1	20.6
Severely obese	28.1	45.4

Source: *International Journal of Obesity*

"Once in college I had a very successful weight loss. The doctor was an older man who gave me some thyroid medicine, and an appetite suppressant. The name of the medicine was Preludin, which you can no longer get in the United States. I was walking all over campus and watching what I was eating. I kept the weight off for a while, but after the break-up from the first romance, I gained the weight back. I was told by a current doctor that it would be medically unethical to prescribe that medicine again. I was very motivated and had pledged to a fraternity. I was looking at all the ladies."

Here is his observation: "Keeping it off is the giant killer."

"When I was a student the exercise was for free. I didn't have to plan to do it. With the little time given between classes, I had to practically run between one class and the next. As an adult, I have to get in the car and go somewhere to exercise."

Henry sent me an advertisement from the 1950s. The store was offering a fall and winter fashion book that was free for "Chubbies." It covered clothes for girls and teens "too chubby to fit into regular sizes." These clothes used to be the half sizes as in 8 ½, 10 ½ through 16 ½.

On my living room end table I keep one of the latest catalogs from a women's plus size store, and I am just waiting for the day when I can contact them to have them take my name off their mailing list. I am already starting to feel less of a "chubby" and more of a "just average."

We finished off the conversation talking about our families. I thanked him for his time and the interview. He said I can feel free to call him for a follow-up if I wish. He is a special man to me, because he has done a lot in the past to help our family.

While I was sitting at Taco Bell eating my low calorie taco, three men walked in. Two were regular height, and one was a good foot and a half taller than the others. I noticed how long and lean his legs were. I was thinking how that could be my friend Henry.

Trucking Away the Fat

Today is garbage pick-up day. I watched as the truck drove up, lifted up the cans, and dumped the trash. I'm thinking, yeah baby, just lift me up and dump out my fat in your big belly and carry it away. Wouldn't it be nice if it were so simple?

I see a skinny lady walk by with her dog. I think, "Look how fast she is walking." Maybe someday with some of my extra pounds deposited to the fat truck, it will be me walking that fast. It all depends on me. It's not the doctor, it's not the class, and it's not the diet books, but it is ME and my mind that will make the ultimate decision.

It was time to leave the house to go to water exercises, where I meet some of my friends. I was curious as to why they came to exercise. One friend is wheelchair bound, so for her, being in the water is a real treat. Another lady who stands close to me in the pool said she used to be a ballerina, and because of doing this for years, her toes and calves are injured. Water exercises are the best exercises for her. An older friend told me she had tendon injuries and she exercises in the pool for fitness and weight control.

I was talking to an Asian man in the pool, asking him the same question. I joked with him saying, "Do you come to the pool to see all the pretty ladies?" He burst into a loud laugh. I was hoping not too many people heard, as I didn't want to have attention drawn in my direction for disrupting the class. Luckily, the instructor wasn't standing next to us, but was down at the other end of the pool. The man's answer was simple. "I like the water." Another man I know told me he was having back problems and his doctor told him to try water exercises before surgery. He no longer needs the surgery.

Peggy S, who once was so kind and came to my home to teach me how to make soap, said, "I come to move, as this is the only exercise I get. I also enjoy talking with the other ladies." This mirrors my sentiments.

For whatever reasons the other people are using the pool, we are all moving, and in one way or another, everyone feels they are benefiting.

I have also added walking to my exercises. Sometimes for a real treat David and I go for a drive. When we get to our destination, we walk and talk. After the danger from the tsunami was over and the waves were only four feet high, we walked above the ocean along West Cliff Drive in Santa Cruz for two hours. We were so happy walking and enjoying the sun's warming rays that it wasn't even "exercise" anymore.

Food Fear Ahead

Articles I read say that you can't let fear get in your way in your efforts to change your behavior. My friend Tammy wrote me an e-mail about going out to eat. I am a little afraid of doing this, as I think this will sabotage my weight loss progress. There will be temptation all around, and I don't know how I am going to handle it.

> Dear Kirsten,
>
> My sentiments exactly: I dread eating out, whether at a restaurant or in another home. What I have learned after two years of practice, is that restaurants will actually do what you tell them to do. They are anxious for your business. I was formerly too shy to ask for something that wasn't specifically on the menu; That has changed for me!
>
> If I know the name of the restaurant where I will be eating, I check out the menu online beforehand. If I have questions about the possibility of getting things done my way, I place a phone call to the restaurant. In the main, I stick with grilled fish (preferably white fish of some sort), shrimp, chicken, or turkey. Add salad - with dressing on the side

or with salsa - and some steamed veggies. I avoid all manner of starch as I know it's not worth the calories. For dessert: Coffee or tea, giving me something to do with my hands and mouth.

If I am eating at the home of someone else, AND if I don't know the hosts very well, I simply pick out the things that I can eat without going wildly over-budget calorie-wise, drink lots of water during the meal, and concentrate on conversation. I avoid pre-dinner snacks (rule of thumb: 100 calories or more per handful or bite), and remove myself from the line of sight of the snack table. Honestly, avoiding eye-contact is an amazingly powerful trick. It is highly effective also at work when well-meaning souls bring in lovely baked goods to share.

I completely agree that there is no such thing as a food holiday: It is the beginning of a slippery slope, and, again, not worth it.

The hardest but most important thing to learn and ACCEPT is that we are not blessed with a "spender" metabolism. We are "savers" and always will be, necessitating a different food intake lifestyle than we are conditioned to want.

I wish you lots and lots of strength.
Sincerely, Tammy

Changing Behavior Is the Answer

Scientific American, February 2011, had an article titled, "How to Fix the Obesity Crisis." It talks about the overweight person wanting to shed pounds quickly, and I'm no different. The situation has to do with part biology, part environment, and part the person's determination to lose weight.

In the magazine, there is a drawing of a human body and it has lines to various parts. The line to the brain says, "The hypothalamus and brain stem help to regulate feelings of hunger and fullness." This is obviously written by a thin scientific type person. I don't know of one overweight person who has issues with being hungry, and that is why they want to eat.

In the article I agree that metabolism and genes play a part in the total design of a person. The one thing that the article says that I really agree with is that, "The most successful way to date to lose at least modest amounts of weight and keep it off with diet and exercise employs programs that focus on changing behavior."

The article talks about four steps to losing weight: (1) the initial assessment; (2) self-monitoring; (3) behavioral shifts; and (4) support groups. Before step one comes the most important step which is self-commitment initiated in the person's own mind. Without this preliminary step, none of the other steps will succeed.

It is the repeating of healthy habits day after day, even on your "terrible" days, that brings success. Even on those terrible days you need to have confidence in yourself, while at the same time being patient to ride out the crisis that threatens to derail you. You are not the employee anymore; you are the manager.

Carrots Instead of Cookies

I am still a nervous eater, especially after lunch and before dinner. My obsession to eat is still there. The only difference is I reach for a carrot instead of a cookie. It is a training exercise. Eventually a student, after practicing the multiplication tables over and over, learns how to do them correctly. The carrot is the correct way for me.

Mountains Will Always Be There

Terrible days will come in our path, just like the "Scientific American" article said. I got a phone call from Kaiser Permanente. I figured it was an appointment reminder for David. My daughter-in-law was on the other end of the phone asking one of us to come and pick up our son. They were in the emergency room because my granddaughter had an allergic reaction. My daughter-in-law asked me to bring some corn syrup to use to camouflage the taste of the crushed pills, which are the real medicine. I checked my pantry as I thought I had some, which I did. Luckily, I began treating the bladder infection that I woke up with early that morning, so that by noon as we drove to the hospital I was already feeling better.

My son was standing outside the emergency room entrance waiting for us. He was holding his infant son, who was so tired that he just gazed into space. If he hadn't been at the hospital, he would have been down for his nap.

As I entered the hospital, the guard had another woman look up what room my little granddaughter was in. They told me room number two. After asking for directions I was on my way, walking a little faster than normal. Actually, I was walking a lot faster than normal.

Here is what I saw when I entered the room. My granddaughter's head and chest were slightly raised because the head of the bed was elevated to a 45 degree angle. Her mother was hovering over her, like a loving mother should. What I saw, underneath the white sheet, looked like the shape of a little bean. Her little red flushed face was all that I could see. She was very still and didn't say a word.

I told her that she was the best angel pie ever, and to take the corn syrup medicine that I brought, because that would make her sweeter, just like angel pie. For one second, just one second, a little smile appeared on her face. Oh, if I had the power I would have made her well right then and there. She would have sat up in the bed and wanted me to read silly poems to her, which both of us enjoy. When I get old, I hope she will read them to me, so we both can laugh again.

My heart ached seeing her this way. I knew her mother and the hospital staff were caring for her, but it BROKE MY HEART to see her like that. It hurt so very bad, as I love that little girl so much. Mechanically I walked down the hall to the hospital exit. We drove my son and grandson home so they could both take a nap.

My thoughts drifted back to my granddaughter most of the day. I broke down and called my son at 3:30 p.m. Everyone had just come home from the hospital. I asked to speak to my little granddaughter to tell her I loved her, but she beat me to it. Her voice was loud and strong when she said, "I LOVE YOU, GRANDMA!" Then she returned to watch the movie they were playing for her. Her voice was like hearing church bells ringing. It was so powerful, not like that little girl lying in the hospital bed. That ill little girl disappeared and I am so happy about that. Another mountain climbed and conquered.

The Diversity of Life

The sorrow of my father's death spurred me on to find the joy of my life, David.

The same foreign travels that excited me also brought me fear.

The same savory foods that brought me joy in preparing and eating, also later knifed me at the scale.

The same Georgia pines that brought me nature's beauty also brought me solitary sadness.

Life is a potpourri of polar opposites, to enjoy when the times are good, and to climb over the mountains when they are difficult.

My life is so much happier now that I am back from Georgia. I am drawn to my grandchildren like a moth is to a flame. They light up my life and warm up my heart. It is the little things that capture my attention. David and I held each one of them up so that they could sit in the apple tree. A smile came on my little two year old grandson's face. When my five year old granddaughter was held up in the tree she pretended to be a bird as she flapped her arms around like she was flying.

After they went home I sat on the sofa smiling: I saw a little blue toy car that had escaped from the clean-up and was ready to drop off the cliff of the tiled hearth into the black ash stained pit of the fireplace. When my little grandson left, he said, "Goodbye dinos [plastic dinosaurs], goodbye trucks." I'm thinking, "Hello, happiness."

When the grandchildren come to visit, my granddaughter shows us her handstands. We play "Wheels on the Bus" over and over for my little grandson, as he loves to dance to this song. Sometimes I wrap one in a fleece blanket to become a burrito, and then I wrap the other. This is called the burrito game. When exhaustion hits, as I am much older, we play the "quiet" game. This is where I say one, two, three, quiet. Then we mimic each other's hand movements to see who can make the other one laugh first.

My latest ritual is the "crunch party." Because eating a lot of finger vegetables has become a way of life for me, I love to offer them this food. I prepare strips of celery, green pepper, baby carrots and pickles, and pass this plate around for all of us to enjoy our "crunch party." The idea started with the sound of the crunch of the carrots. This isn't a baby step for me anymore; it is a gigantic leap.

My Friends on My Virtual Mountain

Climbing down a mountain is hard. As of this date, June 6, 2011, I have lost 46 pounds, just by chip, chip, chipping away at it. On the mountain I had to get enough sleep and drink enough water. It takes hard work and perseverance. Climbing down is not just physical, but it is also mental. Actually, I said that in reverse order. Mental is the most important thing. I knew that before I ever started to descend Mount Everest.

The secret I have discovered over these four months is that I have to turn my food thoughts around 180 degrees, so that food doesn't have the hold on me that it used to. I must stop feeling the sorrow about it, as that is the path back to food. When food no longer becomes an important issue in my life, I can make it all the way down the mountain.

I have to be strong climbing down the mountain, because injuries such as hurting my knee can interfere, but I can't give up. Road blocks, such as birthday parties, always appear.

I want to thank my e-mail support team that climbed down Mount Everest with me. One of the mountain climbing tips is to never climb alone, and I didn't. Maria was by my side singing. Rebecca and Tammy were giving me valuable tips to make my journey successful. Ursula and Yoko both experienced in the pitfalls of climbing walked along with us. The front of the group was held up by Victor and Victoria to defend us from the high calorie invaders. At the very front stood General Bob, who has his age, wisdom and strength to lead the expedition. Sam was walking behind with Edgar, who was pulling the sleds full of supplies.

In my dreams, I wish to see Henry with us. Sam has an extra hiking stick that he will gladly share. How lucky I am to have such a special team walking with me. Sunshine is radiating goodness over all of us. This is one fantastic support team and I thank all of you. As I am walking my backpack has become lighter by 60 pounds.

Tip # 21

"Trust yourself. Create the kind of self that you will be happy to live with all your life. Make the most of yourself by fanning the tiny, inner sparks of possibility into flames of achievement."
–Golda Meir

In navigating the sea of calories, don't let your small boat become a shipwreck.

"The difference between try and triumph is a little umph."
–Author Unknown

Epilogue

While we were on our vacation traveling through central California toward Zion National Park in Utah, we stopped at a gas station/souvenir shop/fast food restaurant all complete in one location. I bought two dinosaur postcards to write brief "I love you" messages to my grandchildren. As I walked past the rows of candy, sodas, bread and canned goods, I spied tables in the fast food section of this highway truck stop. I could use a table to sit down to write my postcards. After I had written them a "food moment" hit me. I wanted something to eat, not because I was hungry, but because always, in my life before, we had always had a piece of pie and a soda or a cup of tea.

Being aware of what was happening to me, I rose up from the chair and told David we had to leave. As I walked away from temptation, my e-mail friends all walked out with me. David understands my struggle, but he is lucky that he doesn't have a weight problem, and he admits he never "loved food" the way I did.

Once in the car I pulled out a bag of celery that I had prepared in the motel room the night before. When getting the celery ready to cut I got a dinner knife from my purse. I have always taken a dinner knife on trips to generously spread peanut butter on sandwiches. I struggled cutting the celery with this dull knife. As I was struggling with it I thought about my struggles with weight. Next time I'll bring a sharper knife, as I have been sharpening up my brain into the new me. I struggled with the celery, but I ultimately succeeded.

At the motel continental breakfast the next morning, I brought my own package of instant oatmeal. The night before all I saw were plastic bins of sugary cereal which I didn't want. As I walked the line around the choices that were available, all I saw were bagels, bread, cream cheese and packets of jelly. I just stared at these choices, realizing this was my old life.

When we pulled off the freeway for lunch at a strip mall, we drove to the shade of a building that housed the Rocky Mountain Chocolate Factory. I didn't dare get out of the car, as that would have been too dangerous. When David cut the submarine sandwich we had brought with us for lunch, I noticed that the knife still had slivers of celery remaining on it, evidence of a quick clean-up job to get on the road again. This was a reminder to me to stay on the celery path, and not to venture off down the Rocky Mountain ice cream road.

The adjacent mall where we went to buy a notebook for me to continue writing had only four non-food stores. I saw the Cold Stone Creamery, Durango's Mexican Grill, Subway, a Japanese restaurant and Red Lobster. The sea of calories was circling around me, and I knew I had to steer myself away from temptation. Before my new lifestyle I never realized how intense the food choices were that we have available to us.

As I was walking in Zion National Park and Bryce Canyon National Park, I remembered that walking in the afternoon just a year ago made my feet ache. Now I had a lightness in my step, and I could actually feel that I was carrying less weight than before. Sixty pounds does make a difference physically. It also makes a wonderful difference mentally, in that I'm re-entering the world of "just being average" again. That feels so good to me, better than chocolate bunnies taste. One feeling can last a long time if you let it, and the other can melt in seconds if you hike in the wrong direction on the mountain.

Tip # 22
"There Are Always Two Choices. Two paths to take. One is easy. And its only reward is that it's easy."
–Unknown

Ecstasy surges through me like water shooting from a fountain. When I began my current weight loss journey I weighed much more than I do today. In desperation I struggled, always keeping focused through the difficulties that lay ahead each pound of the way. Discovering that I have been awarded first prize in the weight loss class brings tears of joy to my eyes. I have learned a new and better way of living.

The journey is not the easy path, but exceedingly worth it. Once I lost those 60 pounds I gained strength, confidence, and courage. Dear Readers, come together with me, and we'll walk as partners to continue down Mount Everest.

Notes

This book is based on e-mail and phone calls, and includes a New Jersey court case.

It contains information I learned at a weight loss class, my personal experiences, and thoughts. All quotes are given author recognition.

My accomplishment of writing this book is due to the many people who participated in my weight loss journey, as well as the special teachers from my weight loss class. The names of all these people have been changed to protect their privacy.

Bibliography

Books/Magazines

Bauman, Ed. "Michelle Obama's Rx for Healthy Kids." *Common Ground.* March 2011: 40.

Buettner, Dan. *"The Secrets of Long Life."* National Geographic. Nov. 2005. Vol. 208: 2-27.

Cloud, John. "*Why Exercise Won't Make You Thin.*" Time. August 17, 2009: Vol. 174, Issue 6. 42-47.

Dawn, Laura, ed. *It Takes A Nation.* 2006. San Rafael, Earth Aware, 20, 94.

Ferguson, Niall. "UN-AMERICAN REVOLUTIONS Most rebellions end in carnage and tyranny. So why are Americans cheering on the Arab wave?" Newsweek. March 7, 2011. Vol.157: 2-3.

Foxx, Richard M. and Azrin, Nathan. *Toilet Training In Less Than A Day.* 1974. New York: Simon Schuster.

Freedman, David H. "How to fix the obesity crisis." *Scientific American.* Feb. 2011. Vol. 304. 40-47.

Friedel, RO, "Dopamine Dysfunction in Borderline Personality Disorder: A Hypothesis," Neuropsychopharmacology. 29: 1029-1039, 2004.

Garmey, Jane. *Great British Cooking: A Well Kept Secret. Over 200 recipes from meat pies to plum pudding – adapted for American cooks.* 1981. New York: Random House, xiii.

Greene, Gayle. *Insomniac.* 2008, Berkeley, Los Angeles, London: University of California Press, 155, 172.

Jacoby, Susan. *Never Say Die.* 2011. New York, Random House, 22.

Jaret, Peter. "*Beating the Urge to Eat.*" Reader's Digest. July 2004: 118.

Keeton, Kathy. *Longevity: The Science Of Staying Young*, Viking Penguin New York, New York 1992. P 271-272, P 136-137, P185-186.

Kidder, Tracy. *Mountains Beyond Mountains: The Quest of Dr. Paul Farmer, a Man Who Would Cure the World.* 2003. New York: Random House, 2.

Web

"Intervention: Dealing With Disordered Eating." *The California Report. Health Dialogues.* PBS. KQED, San Francisco. 24 June 2011. <http://www.californiareport.org/archive/R201102172000/a>

"Nutrition and Toxicity Modulation: The Impact of Animal Body Weight on Study Outcome." International Journal of Toxicology – (February 1998) 17: 1-3. <http://ijt.sagepub.com/content/17/2_suppl/1.extract>

911 Weight Loss. "Human Gene Modification Is The Latest Medical Breakthrough On Obesity." 25 June 2011. <http:/www.911weightloss.org/obesity/human-gene-modification-is-the-latest-medical-breakthrough-on-obesity/>

Barnhard, Neal, MD. "Hooked on Food." MedicineNet.com (22 July 2011). <http://www.medicinenet.com/script/main/art.asp?articlekey=56880>

Forer, Ben "Arizona Governor Proposes Revamping Medicaid Program." April 1, 2011. <http://abcnews.go.com/Health/arizona-gov-jan-brewer-proposes-medicare-fat-fine/story?id=13274368>

Grayson, Mathis and Charlotte, E. "Break Your Food Addictions." Web MD, 19 Feb. 2011. <http://www.webmd.com/diet/features/break-your-food-addictions>

Hartocollis, Anemona. "Rise Seen in Medical Efforts to Treat the Very Old." 18 July 2008. <http://www.nytimes.com/2008/07/18/health/18old.html>

Jensen, Chris. "40 Pounds in 12 Weeks: A Love Story." Theater Review. 9 March, 2011. <http://www.sfweekly.com/2011-03-09/culture/40-pounds-in-12-weeks-a-love-story-theater-review/>

Miko, Francis T. and Froehlich, Christian. "Germany's Role in Fighting Terrorism: Implications for U.S. Policy." CRS Report for Congress, 27 December 2004. <http://www.fas.org/irp/crs/RL32710.pdf>

New Jersey Superior Court, Appellate Division. "Gimello v. Agency Rent-A-Car Systems, Inc." 25 June, 2011. <http://nj.findacase.com/research/wfrmDocViewer.aspx/xq/fac.19910802_0040434.NJ.htm/qx>

Parker-Pope, Tara. "Should Doctors Lecture Patients About Their Weight?" New York Times. 1 July 2008. <http://well.blogs.nytimes.com/2008/07/09/should-doctors-lecture-patients-about-their-weight/>

Salters-Pedneault, Kristalyn, PhD. "Dopamine." About.com (updated August 20, 2008). <http://bpd.about.com/od/glossary/g/dopamine.htm>

Sapolsky, Robert and Michael Meany. "Neuroscience For Kids Newsletter." 4. Stress and Behavior. April 2001. <http://faculty.washington.edu/chudler/news54.html>

Smith, Melinda and Joanna Saisan. "Drug Abuse And Addiction." 22 June 2011. <http://www.helpguide.org/mental/drug_substance_abuse_addiction_signs_effects_treatment.htm>

Wikipedia. "Calorie restriction." 28 July 2011. <http://en.wikipedia.org/wiki/Calorie_restriction>

Wikipedia. "Diet Soda." Wikipedia. 24 June, 2011. <http://en.wikipedia.org/wiki/Diet_soda>

Wikipedia. "Expectancy theory." 25 June 2011. <http://en.wikipedia.org/wiki/Expectancy_theory>

Wikipedia. "Gastric Bypass Surgery." 03 July, 2011. <http://en.wikipedia.org/wiki/Gastric_bypass_surgery>

Wikipedia. "Heart Rate." 22 June 2011. <http://en.wikipedia.org/wiki/Heart_rate_>

About Kirsten Crabill

Kirsten Crabill is a housewife and mother of two children. She studied elementary education at The University of Maryland, and is the author of unpublished journals on England, China and Indonesia.

She lives with her husband in the San Francisco Bay Area.

Made in the USA
Charleston, SC
30 November 2011